Radiography

An Introduction to Diagnostic Radiography

P. H. Carter
FCR, TDCR, CertEd
Principal, The North Trent School of
Diagnostic Radiography, Sheffield

Churchill Livingstone ▦

EDINBURGH LONDON MELBOURNE AND NEW YORK 1984

CHURCHILL LIVINGSTONE
Medical Division of Longman Group Limited

Distributed in the United States of America by Churchill Livingstone Inc., 1560 Broadway,
New York, N.Y. 10036, and by associated companies, branches and representatives
throughout the world.

© Longman Group Limited 1984

First published 1984

ISBN 0 443 02880 X

British Library Cataloguing in Publication Data
Carter, P. H.
    An introduction to diagnostic radiography.
    1. Diagnosis, Radioscopic
    I. Title
    616.07′57   RC78

Library of Congress Cataloging in Publication Data
Carter, P. H. (Peter H.)
    An introduction to diagnostic radiography.
    Includes index.
    1. Diagnosis, Radioscopic,   I. Title.
RC78.C38 1984   616.07′572   83-15356

Printed in Singapore by
Selector Printing Co (Pte) Ltd.

Preface

The learning opportunities offered to a student radiographer within an X-ray department, are immense — and of vital importance. But X-ray departments are busy places. A newcomer is easily bewildered by the equipment, procedures and work flow. Students have difficulty in identifying their learning needs and, at first, in finding the courage to ask questions.

During this early stage, supervising radiographers, both clinical and in schools, have a problem too. Each student's learning pattern is shaped by individual circumstances and attitudes. This variety can make it difficult to plan formal instruction — will it be too soon or too late, too simple or too complicated?

The attitudes formed during a student's introductory weeks and months may have permanent significance. If learning needs are satisfied, one step leads to another and a student is encouraged to ask further questions. An inquisitive attitude is valuable, if not essential, in establishing a successful career.

On the other hand, if students' needs remain unsatisfied — through either absence of help or untimely preoccupation with less relevant topics — the habit of enquiring fails to develop. Learning then becomes, and may remain, a struggle.

This book has been compiled as an offer of help to students, new to diagnostic radiography. It has a question-and-answer framework within which can be found some basic explanations and facts about radiography. More than this, however, it is offered as a stimulus to the development of positive attitudes: to look for learning potential in every situation; to develop practical and intellectual skills; to regard all work as a challenge; and to enjoy it!

Sheffield, 1984

P.H.C.

Acknowledgements

I am grateful to a large number of colleagues who, over many years, have shared their experience and attitudes with me. Their influence has helped to form the outlook and philosophy which underlie this book.

The diagrams which the reader will find such an important help to understanding the text are the work of Mr Patrick M. Elliott.

Much credit for the appearance of this book must go to Messrs Churchill Livingstone, who have been encouraging and unfailingly helpful throughout its production.

Final preparation of the manuscript would not have been possible without the help of Mrs June Elliott, with assistance from Mrs Jenny Pearson and Mrs Margaret Law.

Lastly, I must thank my wife, Sheila, and children, Helen and Nicholas, for putting up with the disruptions for which this book was responsible.

P.H.C.

Contents

Glossary of Radiographic Terms

Anode	A positively-charged electrode. Most relevant in radiography with reference to that part of an X-ray tube at which X-rays are produced.
Artefact	A thing which does not occur naturally. The term is used to describe features of a radiographic image which are accidental inclusions and not parts of the patient's body.
Bucky	A moving, secondary radiation grid assembly; named in honour of its inventor.
Cathode	A negatively-charged electrode. Relevant in radiography mainly as the X-ray tube electrode at which the electron beam is produced. Also, in an electrolytic silver recovery assembly, the electrode at which metallic silver is deposited.
Caudad	Term used when the X-ray beam is angled away from its normal 90° relationship to the film. Literally means 'towards the tail' but can also describe a downward angulation towards the foot, when a lower limb is radiographed.
Cephalad	Term used when the X-ray beam is angled away from its normal 90° relationship to the film. Literally means 'towards the head': thus confusion can arise during skull radiography, unless a more specific description — e.g., 'towards the vertex' is used.
Collimate	Term used with reference to an X-ray beam to indicate a restriction of its dimensions.
Compression	Pressure applied to a part of the patient's body, by means of a fabric band or plastic shell, to displace movable tissue away from a specific area of interest, enabling it to be shown more clearly.

Cone	A metal cylinder which can be attached to an X-ray tube with the purpose of producing a fixed, limited X-ray field, and possibly assisting in tube positioning.
Contrast	The difference between photographic densities on a radiographic image. Can refer to either a whole image, when it describes the range from highest to lowest densities, or a specific feature against the background of its adjoining structures.
Contrast agent	A substance of either high effective atomic number or low density, introduced into an object to enhance its contrast for the duration of a radiographic examination.
Contrast medium	An alternative term for a contrast agent. (Students should note that confusion can arise between the singular form, *medium*, and incorrect use of the plural, *media*).
Density	Term used in either of two senses: (i) Photographically, density describes precisely the degree of blackening of a given area of a radiographic image. It is the logarithmic ratio between the light intensities incident on, and transmitted through, a radiograph. (ii) In a physical sense, it is a measure of the mass per unit volume of a substance, and is a factor in determining its radiopacity.
Field	Area exposed by an X-ray beam.
Filter	A selective barrier. Relevant in two contexts: with reference to X-rays, it is a thin plate (usually of aluminium) used to remove low-energy radiation from the beam; in a darkroom safelight, it is a coloured glass plate which removes the shorter wavelength visible light from the 'white' light emitted by an electric lamp.
Fluorography	The technique of recording a radiographic image solely by the action of light from a fluorescent screen — i.e., there is no exposure of the film to X-rays. A camera is used with an optical system which reduces the image to a miniature size.
Fluoroscopy	The technique of *watching* an object on a fluorescent screen, under X-ray control. The screen is viewed via an image intensifier and closed-circuit television system.
Focal spot	The small, defined area of the X-ray tube anode, bombarded by electrons from the filament, and from which X-rays are emitted.
Focus	An alternative term for the focal spot of an X-ray tube.
Fog	An undesirable photographic density superimposed on an image. It can originate from accidental exposure to X-rays or safelighting or be a sign of 'stale' film or faulty processing conditions. Its effect is to increase lower image densities, while having much less effect on the higher densities. It thus reduces image contrast.
Generator	The part of an X-ray equipment assembly which supplies and controls the power to the X-ray tube.

Grid	A metallic lattice, designed to permit *controlled* transmission. The term is most commonly used to describe a device placed between object and film to eliminate scattered radiation from the X-ray beam, with the purpose of enhancing image contrast. Also a device to control passage of electrons across an X-ray tube.
Irradiate	Expose to radiation. (*Irradiation* also describes the light scattering which occurs within film and intensifying screens when a radiograph is exposed, leading to photographic unsharpness.)
Kilovolt (*kV*)	One thousand (10^3) volts. The unit in which the potential difference across a diagnostic X-ray tube is measured.
Markers	Radiopaque letters and numerals affixed to the front of an X-ray film or cassette to record information permanently on a radiograph.
Milliampere (*mA*)	One thousandth (10^{-3}) of an ampere. The unit in which the current through an X-ray tube is measured.
Milliampere second (*mAs*)	The product of tube current (mA) and exposure time (measured in seconds). A unit of electric charge equal to a millicoulomb.
Photon	A small, discrete quantity or 'package' of radiation.
Primary X-radiation	X-radiation originating from the focal spot of an X-ray tube.
Projection	A radiographic image produced when the X-ray beam is directed through the object in a specified manner. Students should note that a projection is independent of the patient's position (whether prone, supine or erect, for example) although the radiographic appearance of the object may well be influenced by the position.
Quantum	An alternative term for a photon.
Radiograph	Concerning the production of an image through the action of X-rays, this term refers both to the procedure and to the resulting image. (Corresponds to 'photograph' when an image is created by visible light.)
Radiolucent	Permitting relatively easy transmission of X-rays.
Radiopaque	Offering (discernible) opposition to the transmission of X-rays.
Resolution	The ability of an image recording system to resolve, or record the detail contained within, an incident pattern of light or X-rays. Expressed quantitatively in line pairs per millimetre.
Safelighting	Visible light of a restricted range of wavelengths (colours) to which specified film or other photographic material is relatively insensitive.
Scattered X-rays	X-radiation which is diverted from its original path by interaction with matter.
Screening	A colloquial term for fluoroscopy. It derives from the original technique in which, before the use of image intensification and television, the image was produced on a simple fluoroscopic screen and viewed in a totally

darkened room. (Students should note that this term has a wider, medical meaning: the examination of a large number of people for evidence of a specific disease.)

Secondary X-radiation

X-rays emitted or scattered from matter exposed to a primary X-ray beam.

Tomography

A technique which produces an image of a *slice* through an object, rather than of its whole. The term refers to both conventional imaging techniques and to computed image reconstruction (computed tomography).

Unsharpness

Blurring of image detail. No radiographic image is considered to be free from the causes of unsharpness, notably the fact that the X-ray tube focal spot is not a point source. Since absolute sharpness is thus unobtainable, it is customary to refer to greater or lesser degrees of unsharpness.

X-ray

A colloquial term used as a substitute for 'radiograph'.

X-rays

The short-wavelength electromagnetic radiation produced by an X-ray tube.

An Introduction to Diagnostic Radiography

1

What are X-rays?

It is difficult to describe, in a conventional manner, something which is invisible. The fact that X-rays are a form of *electromagnetic radiation* (Fig. 1) may not be significant to all students. It will be helpful, however, to consider some of the *properties* of X-rays.

Penetration. X-rays can penetrate through a structure to varying degrees, depending on the structure's composition.

Other electromagnetic radiations are able to penetrate. Radio waves, for example, pass easily through walls, to reach

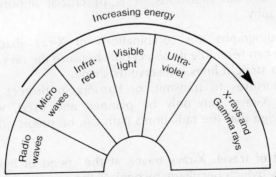

Increasing energy

Radio waves — Micro waves — Infrared — Visible light — Ultraviolet — X-rays and Gamma rays

Fig. 1 The electromagnetic spectrum. X-rays and gamma rays only differ in their origins: X-rays are produced when electrons undergo a change in motion; gamma rays are emitted from radioactive materials.

receivers within buildings. The parts of a structure being radiographed, however, oppose or permit the passage of an X-ray beam, to a *very finely varied degree*. This property forms the foundation of diagnostic radiography.

Photographic effect. In common with some other electromagnetic radiations, X-rays have a *photographic effect*: they can form an image on film. Photographic film has been the principal medium for recording radiographic images over the years since the discovery of X-rays.

Fluorescence. X-rays were discovered by Professor W. C. Roentgen in 1895. Leading directly to their discovery was the property of being able to cause *fluorescence*.

Certain chemicals, termed *phosphors*, emit ultraviolet radiation and visible light when exposed to, or 'excited by' X-rays. This property figures very importantly in the diagnostic applications of X-rays in medicine:

1. A fluorescent *screen* is used for procedures which involve watching movements of, or manipulation of an object. This technique is termed *'fluoroscopy'*.
2. A form of fluorescence, *'scintillation'*, may be employed to detect and measure X-rays, in computed tomography equipment.
3. X-ray film is usually exposed, tightly sandwiched between a pair of fluorescent *intensifying screens*, within a cassette.

Rectilinear propagation. This property, of travelling *in straight lines* diverging from the source, is a feature of all electromagnetic radiations. It is of crucial importance in radiography:

1. Radiographs are combinations of X-ray shadows. A shadow can resemble its object only because the rays, by travelling in straight lines, preserve its shape.
2. Apertures to transmit, or barriers to protect persons against X-rays, can only be planned and used, with the knowledge that the radiation's path can be predicted, in this way.

Speed of travel. X-rays travel 'at the speed of light'. This property (which peculiarly recognises the commonest form of electromagnetic radiation) tends to be taken for granted, but it has some importance:

1. When the exposure button is pressed, an object is instantaneously recorded in its state and position.

2. The immediate X-ray hazards disappear at the end of an exposure — no residual radiation lurks around afterwards!

Intensity variation with distance. It is to be expected that the intensity of an X-ray beam becomes less, as the measuring point is moved further and further away from the radiation source. In common with other electromagnetic radiations, if emitted from a point source (or nearly so): X-radiation intensity reduces according to the *squared value* of the increasing distance between source and measuring point (assuming there is no interposed absorbing medium). Similarly, if this distance is reduced, intensity is observed to increase — again, with the squared value of the distance. By this fact, X-rays are said to obey an *Inverse Square Law*.

1. This must be borne in mind if, when a patient is about to be radiographed, the distance between the X-ray tube and the film needs to be altered.

2. If a radiographer is unable to shelter behind the usual, large lead screen at the moment of making an exposure — in an operating theatre, perhaps, or in a hospital ward — it is important to remember that intensity is significantly reduced by an increase in the distance separating the radiographer from the source of radiation. In other words, even if a protective apron is being worn, it is wise to stand well back!

Ionisation. Exposure to X-rays cannot be immediately detected by any of the human senses. This fact is reassuring to a nervous patient anticipating pain but takes on an entirely different significance when a further property, ionisation, is considered. X-rays are able to ionise material — i.e., to split atoms into their constituent negative and positive ions.

If the irradiated (exposed) material is inanimate, the ions normally recombine in their original state. If living cells are exposed to X-rays, however, ionisation can lead to *biological changes*. In patients undergoing radiotherapy, these changes have been calculated and planned, and are intended to be beneficial. In diagnostic radiography, however, such biological changes are wholly undesired and must be minimised.

In all procedures which involve radiation, there is a need to avoid accidental exposure of personnel — whether patients or staff. The possible biological consequences of exposure to radiation explain this need. But the fact that X-rays *cannot be detected* by a person receiving an exposure, is also of practical importance. An X-ray room door carelessly left open during an exposure, and a patient's companion being allowed to sit within range of an X-ray beam, are examples of dangerous practice which the student must learn to avoid.

Suggested exercises

— The properties of X-rays employed in diagnostic radiography, can be seen every day in the X-ray department.
— Additionally, students may like to see a demonstration of fluorescence, by exposure of an intensifying screen to X-rays (with the cassette open) in a darkened room.
— If two or more types of screen (phosphors) are available, it may be of interest to compare their visible emissions.

Related studies

The general nature and properties of electromagnetic radiations; the inverse square law; physical details of how fluorescence, ionisation and photographic exposure (the latent image) occur.

2

How are X-rays produced?

X-rays are produced when *electrons travelling at very high speeds suddenly undergo a change in motion*. This is made to happen in an X-ray tube — and will be understood more easily if the construction of a tube is described simultaneously.

With reference to Figure 2: within an X-ray tube lies a **cathode** (*C*) which incorporates a **filament** heated by an electric current. Heat causes electrons to be emitted from the filament. These are made to travel across to a clearly defined area of the **anode** (*A*) termed the **target**. Three factors ensure this:

1. *A very high electrical potential difference* is applied between the cathode (–) and anode (+). In diagnostic radiography, this is usually within the range 50 kV to 130 kV. Being negatively charged, electrons are repelled by the cathode and attracted to the anode, reaching it with very high *kinetic energy*.

2. The filament is *recessed* in a concave part of the cathode, termed the **focusing cup**. By repulsion (between like charges) it shapes the electron beam to impinge precisely onto the target.

3. The electrodes are sealed in a glass **envelope** (*E*) which contains a **vacuum** (*V*). The functions of the vacuum include allowing electrons to travel freely from filament to target.

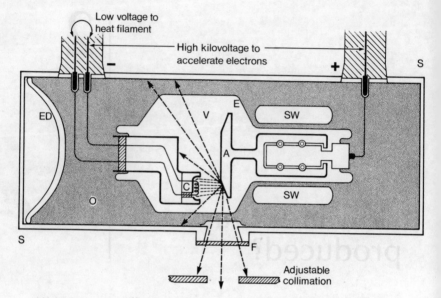

Fig. 2 A rotating anode X-ray tube. Key: (A) anode; (C) cathode; (E) envelope; (V) vacuum; (SW) stator windings; (O) oil; (ED) expansion diaphragm; (F) aluminium filter; (S) shield.

Of the electrons from the filament which bombard the target, *only about 5% have their kinetic energy converted into X-rays*. The remainder of the electrons merely cause the target atoms to vibrate — i.e., their kinetic energy is converted into *heat*. Thus, as a producer of X-rays, the X-ray tube cannot be regarded as an efficient device.

There are two processes by which X-rays are produced:

1. If an electron from the filament passes close to the nucleus of a target atom, it may be deflected from its course by the effect of the nuclear charge (positive acting on negative). The deflection causes a **photon** (a discrete quantity or package) of X-radiation to be produced. Having thus lost energy, the electron slows down but may continue to take part in further reactions.

X-ray tube targets are normally made of the metal, **tungsten**. In addition to its favourable physical properties (including a very high melting point), tungsten has a high atomic number (74) — that is, a highly positive nuclear charge. It is thus an efficient element for producing X-rays.

As this process slows down the electrons, the X-rays so produced are known as '*braking radiation*' (or, in German, 'Bremsstrahlung'). The photons of radiation may have any amount of energy (depending on the original kinetic energy of the electron and the violence with which it reacts with the target nucleus) up to a maximum value, related to the peak potential difference applied across the X-ray tube. They form a 'continuous spectrum'.

2. Alternatively, an incident electron can collide with one of the electrons orbiting an atomic nucleus. If its kinetic energy is greater than the binding energy of the orbiting electron, the collision ejects this electron, creating a vacancy.

The filling of this vacancy occurs in a particular manner. An electron from an outer orbit (i.e., further away from the nucleus) comes very quickly in and, in doing so, loses a *precise* amount of energy — which is emitted as a photon of X-radiation.

Since the energy of such photons is determined by the energy differences between orbits (or 'shells') in the atoms of the particular element, the term '*characteristic radiation*' is used.

X-rays travel from the target *in all directions*. Those directed inwards are effectively absorbed within the anode, but from the face of the target emerges a beam which approaches coverage of a hemisphere. Of this, only a small segment is used: the rays which travel in the direction of and through the X-ray tube's **window**. Having passed through a **filter** (F) the beam's cross-sectional area is further restricted by **collimation**, usually with lead diaphragms, to the size required.

The unused majority of X-radiation emitted from the face of the target represents a potential hazard to patients and staff. The degree to which it is allowed to leak from the X-ray tube must, therefore, be absolutely minimal. This condition is achieved by a *lead lining* within the tube **shield** (S).

The potential difference (**kilovoltage**) applied across the X-ray tube is varied according to circumstances. The main purpose in selecting a kV value is to produce X-radiation having a certain *penetrating power*, but radiation intensity is also affected. The current through the X-ray tube (measured in **milliamperes**) is varied as required, to control radiation *intensity*.

Mention was made earlier of the heat created by the majority of electrons when they bombard the target. This by-product has an enormous influence on X-ray tube design — the aim being to restrict as much as possible, the temperature rise which it causes during an exposure.

The target's angulation is a compromise between the opposing needs to have (a) a *large* area bombarded by the electrons, to minimise temperature rise, and (b) a *small* X-ray source to reduce image unsharpness (effect of penumbra).

In fact, these areas must be identical, since electron bombardment produces X-rays, but angulation *foreshortens the appearance of the area*, when it is 'viewed' through the tube window. Figure 3 shows this relationship. The **true** (or **actual**) **focal area** is the *oblong* area bombarded by electrons and from which X-rays emanate. The **effective** (or **apparent**) **focal area** is the apparently *square* area from which — as far as the image is concerned — X-rays are effectively emitted.

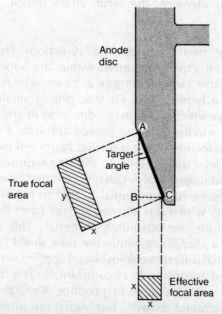

Fig. 3 Relative sizes of true and effective focal areas. BC equals the width of the true focal area and the side length of the square effective focal area. AC is the length of the true focal area. The sine of the target angle = $\dfrac{BC}{AC} = \dfrac{\text{effective}}{\text{true}}$ focal areas.

The relationship between true and effective focal areas depends on the **target** (or **anode**) **angle**. The two areas have a common width but vary in length, with the *sine* of the target angle. Reduction of the target angle makes the ratio between effective and true focal areas more favourable but also reduces achievable field sizes at distances from the target. This is due to the beam 'cut-off', at the target face.

The quoted '**focal spot size**' of an X-ray tube is the *effective focal area*, measured or projected along the *central axis* of the X-ray beam passing through the tube window. (If measured at points away from this central ray, the shape and size of the effective focal area will be different: towards the anode, it will appear foreshortened to a smaller area; towards the cathode, it will seem larger.)

The target of a stationary (or fixed) anode X-ray tube is a rectangular tungsten block, embedded in the sloping surface of a cylindrical copper anode. In a rotating anode tube, it is a rectangular area, aligned with the tube filament, on the angled face of a tungsten disc (see Fig. 4). During exposures, the disc is rotated at high speed — the anode **rotor** assembly and its surrounding **stator windings** (SW) forming an electric motor. Rotation causes rapid and continuous renewal of the bombarded surface. This spreads out the heat along a circular path, rather than restricting it to the rectangular target area alone. Thus the

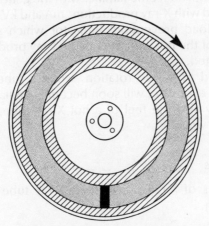

Fig. 4 The face of a rotating anode disc. The shaded rectangle shows the area of the circular focal track which is bombarded by electrons from the tube's filament.

temperature rise of the target area is minimised, for a given amount of heat.

The space between the tube **insert** (the envelope and electrodes) and the shield is filled with **oil** (O) the volume of which is allowed to vary, with temperature, by a flexible **expansion diaphragm** (ED). As well as being an *electrical insulator*, the oil *convects* heat from the insert to the tube shield, from where it is dispersed by air convection.

If the temperature of the *whole* X-ray tube rises dangerously high, the expansion diaphragm can operate a microswitch to cut off the tube's power supply and prevent further exposures until cooling has occurred.

Suggested exercises

The X-ray tube is central to all radiographic equipment; careful study of its construction and operation is important.

— Students should have access to parts of dismantled X-ray tubes, and possibly to a working model of a tube.

— An X-ray tube's outward appearance can be related to its internal construction; students should, for instance, be able to identify the position of the target.

— Students must become familiar with the generator controls concerned with X-ray production: mA and kV selectors and the 'overload prevention' indicator which shows when, because of the heating, the rate of X-ray production has to be restricted.

— The sound of anode rotation, when a tube is prepared before an exposure, will soon become familiar to a student — as may also the feel of a hot X-ray tube, after a busy period of work!

Related studies

The processes of X-ray production; X-ray tube construction and operation.

3

How are radiographic images produced?

When X-rays pass through a patient's body, *shadows* are created. These are invisible, of course, so they differ from shadows cast by everyday objects in the path of visible light. But there is another, important difference. A person standing in sunlight casts a shadow which shows the outlined shape of the *whole* body — because light cannot penetrate: it is either absorbed by or reflected from the body's surface. X-rays, however, since they pass *through* a patient's body, create shadows of the various *structures within* the body.

The beam of X-radiation emerging from a patient's body thus forms a complicated pattern of many shadows — some side-by-side, others overlapping or superimposed; some prominent, others faint.

It is important to understand why some structures are revealed by X-rays more clearly than others. Why, for instance, are skeletal parts of the body more prominent on radiographs than soft tissues and other organs of the body?

Three features of its composition may cause a structure to contrast with its surroundings:

Density

Interactions between X-rays and matter involve the *atoms* of

11

the material under consideration. The lower its density, the fewer are the atoms in a given volume of material. The likelihood that photons of radiation passing into a volume of material will be **attenuated** (i.e. stopped from continuing along their original paths), *increases with the material's density*.

Air and collections of other gases within the body can be shown on radiographs (as darker shades) because their densities are less than those of surrounding solid or liquid structures.

Effective atomic number

Atomic number (i.e. the number of protons in the nucleus or, equally, the number of electrons surrounding it) is a feature unique to each element. The term *'effective'* represents the fact that body tissues contain several different elements. Their combined effect depends not only on the average of the atomic numbers but also on the proportions in which the elements are combined.

The *higher* the effective atomic number, the *greater* is the degree of X-ray attenuation.

The skeleton may readily be seen on a radiograph because bone is relatively dense, but also because it contains calcium (atomic number 20) which raises the effective atomic number to a value twice as great as that for muscle and fat.

Thickness

If an object is homogeneous in terms of its density and effective atomic number, its thicker parts will attenuate X-radiation more than its thinner parts.

The term **radiolucent** is used to describe a structure which (because it has a low density or a low effective atomic number, or simply because it is thin) attenuates X-radiation to only a slight degree. Structures which attenuate X-rays more effectively may be termed **radiopaque**.

Invisible X-ray shadows, carrying information about the patient, may be transformed into visible images by:

1. Using *photographic film*, in which changes are caused by exposure to X-rays.

2. Employing the *fluorescent* effect of X-rays:

a. A pair of fluorescent *intensifying screens* can be used in combination with an X-ray film (usually in a cassette).

b. When it is required to watch the *movement* of structures within the body, a fluorescent screen can be 'viewed' electronically and its image displayed on a television monitor. This technique is termed *fluoroscopy*.

c. A screen image can be photographed and miniaturised on film via an optical system within a *fluorographic camera*.

3. Using other electronic techniques, some involving a computer.

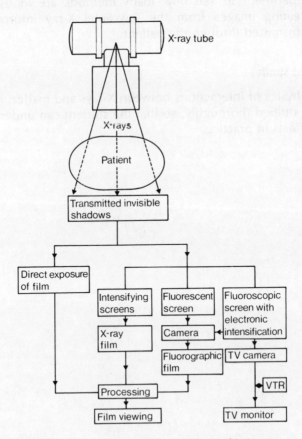

Fig. 5 Conventional methods of producing a radiographic image.

Exposure alone creates no visible effect on an X-ray film; it must subsequently be *processed* to create a permanent, visible image.

Figure 5 summarises these options.

Suggested exercises

— A range of radiographs should be studied, with a view to determining which features of their composition have enabled the various structures to be shown.
— A survey should be made of the equipment in the X-ray department to see how many methods are in use for creating images from the (invisible) X-ray information transmitted through the patient.

Related studies

The physics of interactions between X-rays and matter, needs to be studied thoroughly, so that the student can understand the effects in practice.

4

How does X-ray film differ from ordinary photographic film?

If a student has any knowledge at all, of the film used in an ordinary camera, one point of difference between this and X-ray film, will be obvious — its size. There is a reason for this, and it will be useful to consider the other points of difference, in the same way — through their reasons.

But first, there is an important *similarity*. All types of film incorporate a chemical which is sensitive to light and other, high energy radiations, including X-rays. Three of the elements known as 'halogens', chlorine, bromine and iodine, form compounds which serve this purpose. These **silver halides** are used in the form of minute *crystals* suspended in a very thin layer of *gelatin*, termed an **emulsion**.

Figure 6 shows X-ray film compared with conventional photographic film. The main differences between the two are as follows:

Size

Unlike visible light, X-rays *cannot be focused*. Because of this, radiographs are 'life-sized' — or, in fact, a little larger, since the X-ray beam *diverges* as it travels through the object.

(It should be mentioned that a particular type of X-ray image can be recorded on small-format film. This occurs when the

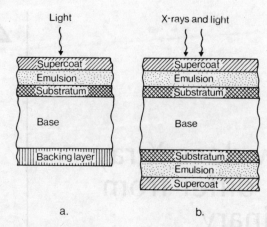

Fig. 6 Cross-sections of (a) photographic (fluorographic) film; and (b) X-ray film.

image on a fluorescent screen is, literally, photographed by a fluorographic camera.)

Two emulsions

A photograph is recorded when light reflected or otherwise emitted from the object, is focused on to and absorbed by a film emulsion. Light approaches the film from one direction only, so a single emulsion is sufficient for the purpose.

Compared with visible light, however, absorption of X-rays by a film emulsion is much less efficient — only a small percentage of the beam's energy is absorbed, the remainder passing through and being virtually wasted. Thus, if *film alone* is used to record a radiograph, there is a proportionately *low efficiency* in the conversion of invisible X-ray information into a visible image.

All types of film have a specified degree of *sensitivity* to the exposing radiation (light, X-rays, etc.). This property is termed '**speed**'; films may be '*slow*' or '*fast*'.

One limited solution to the problem of low energy absorption by film lies in the use of fast film. Photographic film speed is normally dependent on the *size of silver halide grains* and *thickness of the emulsion*. These factors also apply to X-ray film, but there is an additional feature — the *two emulsions*, one on each side of the base, create so-called '**duplitized**' film. The two emulsions increase film speed without reducing the rate at which processing solutions may penetrate; they also tend to prevent a film from curling when wet (one of the functions of ordinary film's backing layer) and, incidentally, make handling easier as there is no 'front' or 'back'.

But the major benefit of duplitized film is the facility to use a pair of *intensifying screens* — and the reader will probably have observed that this is the usual method of exposing radiographs. To describe their action, in brief: intensifying screens greatly *increase* the amount of energy absorbed from the X-ray beam. They pass most of this on to the film in the form of efficiently-absorbed ultra-violet and visible light. Thus, the image-forming effect of X-radiation is considerably intensified.

Colour sensitivity

An 'ordinary photographic film' is usually, today, one which will produce photographs in colour. Radiographs are in black-and-white, so there is obviously a difference between the two types of film in this respect. It is not always appreciated, however, that even black-and-white camera film is sensitive to all colours of visible light — 'panchromatic'. (It needs to be to translate all colours into proportional shades of grey).

A silver halide emulsion is normally sensitive to only the shorter wavelengths of visible light — blue and violet — and to ultra-violet radiation. Sensitivity is extended to other colours, as required, by special treatment during manufacturing.

The colour sensitivity required of X-ray film is determined by the light emitted from intensifying screens: this may be blue/violet, in which case only a basic silver halide ('**monochromatic**') emulsion is needed; or green — when emulsion with an extended sensitivity ('**orthochromatic**') must be used.

Other similarities. (1) Both ordinary and X-ray film have surfaces which are given a degree of protection against contamination and abrasion by a clear, gelatin **supercoating**. (2) The film **base**, in both cases, is a thin, clear, flexible plastic. (3) The emulsions are attached to the film base by an *adhesive substratum*.

Suggested exercises

— The various sizes of X-ray film (cassettes) must be learned by students.
— A sheet of 'scrap' X-ray film should be inspected. A torn edge of this, viewed through an enlarging lens, will reveal the basic layer construction.

Related studies

A detailed look at the construction of X-ray and fluorographic film, including the various types of emulsion that are in use.

5

Why are intensifying screens used?

Students newly-arrived in the X-ray department soon note that Intensifying screens are used for practically all conventional radiographic exposures. This being so, screens must offer some important benefits. These are derived from the fact that intensifying screens *absorb much more energy from an X-ray beam than can be absorbed by a film alone*; and pass this energy to the film in the form of ultraviolet radiation and visible light which the film can absorb with relative efficiency.

Figure 7 shows the construction of an intensifying screen. In use, an X-ray film is sandwiched between a pair of screens. At the moment of exposure, X-radiation passes through both screens, causing fluorescence. This light exposes both film emulsions exactly according to the pattern of X-rays transmitted through the object.

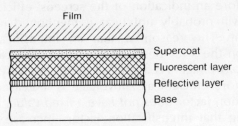

Fig. 7 Cross-section of an intensifying screen.

The **fluorescent layer** is a suspension of a chemical, termed a *phosphor*, in the form of very fine crystals. This layer is bonded on to a strong, flexible plastic **base** which may have a pigmented surface to act as a **reflective layer**. The outer surface of the fluorescent layer is protected by a very thin varnish **supercoat**.

Energy absorbed by film and screens from the X-ray beam transmitted through an object represents information retrieved before the beam passes on to an unproductive final attenuation. The more efficient this retrieval, it follows that the original quantity of radiation necessary to produce the image can be reduced proportionately.

To express this, in terms of *speed*: a film/screen combination is considerably faster than a film alone. This increased speed promotes two important advantages:

1. The smaller quantity of X-rays needed for producing a given radiographic image, presents a **lesser radiation hazard** to the patient.

2. Assuming that the quantity of radiation is reduced by a shortening of the exposure's duration, the **risk of movement during the exposure is lessened.**

There are further implications of these points, for students to learn and discuss during their training. Some of these will now be outlined.

Relative speed

The term **intensification factor** expresses the ratio between two quantities of radiation: the relative *large* quantity required to produce an image *without* the help of intensifying screens, and the much *smaller* quantity when *a given type of screen is used*. It is therefore an indication of the screens' efficiency — but students will probably not hear it mentioned in the X-ray department. The reason is that an intensification factor depends on the X-ray beam quality or, in practical terms, on the *tube kilovoltage*. As a general trend, intensifying screens become more efficient as kilovoltage is increased: thus the intensification factor *does not have a fixed value*.

Assuming that intensification factors increase at approximately the same rate, it is more useful to refer to the **relati-**

ve speed of a pair of intensifying screens — i.e., to compare it with the speed of another type. So, for example, one type may be said to be one-and-a-half times or twice as fast as another type.

Different types of screen

It has been mentioned that different types of intensifying screen have differing speeds. Such differences may be due to the *type* of phosphor; to the *size* of the phosphor crystals; or to the *thickness* of the fluorescent layer. (Speed increases with crystal size and with fluorescent layer thickness.)

Availability of different speeds, might puzzle a student. After all, if intensifying screens bring the benefits of reducing exposure time and reducing radiation hazard to the patient, surely the faster the better?

The answer is, simply, that increased intensifying screen speed cannot be achieved without the risk of lowering another

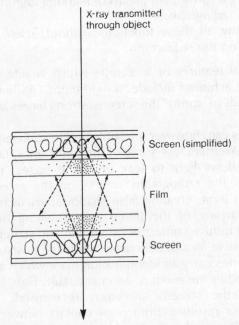

Fig. 8 Response of intensifying screens to an X-ray exposure. Light divergence and scattering increase the affected areas of the film emulsions.

aspect of image quality. The effect of a fluorescing crystal upon the film, is greater in area than the crystal itself, due to the spread of light and subsequent reflection and scattering (see Fig. 8). These effects, diffusing the radiation pattern, may under some circumstances be observable on the radiograph as a form of **photographic unsharpness**.

There are *other* potential causes of image unsharpness, however, which fast intensifying screens *can help to minimise*.

Use of cassettes

Intensifying screens are usually, but not exclusively, used in **cassettes**. It is therefore appropriate to consider briefly the functions and uses of a cassette:

— acting as a *lightproof* holder, to protect the film;
— providing *physical protection* for the intensifying screens;
— keeping the film and intensifying screens in the *closest possible contact*;
— offering a convenient means of marking *identification data* on the radiograph;
— achieving all these functions *without, itself, casting an image* on the radiograph.

Structural features of a cassette which enable these functions to be achieved include: a rigid **frame**, tightly-fitting **back**, **pressure pads** to 'spring' the screens, strong **hinges** and **fastening clips**.

Cassettes can, however, be subjected to sufficient 'wear and tear' to make them lose some of their efficiency. Loss of light-proofing allows light to leak in at the edges, fogging the margins of the radiographs; marks on the screens absorb fluorescent light, creating false shadows, **artefacts**, on radiographs; warping of the frame and spraining of clips and hinges can reduce contact between film and screens. This last fault can cause *localised* increases in image unsharpness.

All cassettes carry an identification mark which allows them to be traced in the event of an image fault. Light leakage and marks on the screens are easily recognised. The image unsharpness resulting from poor contact between film and screens is less easily recognisable — set, as it may be, against a background of unsharpness arising from other causes.

Fortunately, a simple test can confirm or disprove this condition. It involves radiographing a suitable test object (a flat, rigid wire mesh or grid) under conditions in which other causes of unsharpness are either eliminated or reduced to a negligible level.

Radiation protection

Since exposure of the patient to X-rays presents a potential hazard, it would seem natural for the fastest intensifying screens available, to be used on all occasions. But the radiographer has another responsibility to the patient — to produce radiographs from which the patient's condition can be diagnosed. If the image quality obtainable when using the fastest screens falls short of providing sufficient diagnostic information, the choice may fall on slightly slower screens which will satisfy the diagnostician — even though the radiation hazard to the patient will be higher.

Exceptions to the use of intensifying screens

It may prove helpful to look at some instances when intensifying screens are not used:

Extremities. Radiography of the extremities — hand, forearm, foot, ankle, for example — may be undertaken in some X-ray departments, using *direct exposure* of the film to X-rays. The reasoning, in these cases, is that successful diagnosis may depend on demonstration of structures within the object which are so fine that screens could introduce enough unsharpness to conceal them.

This practice, of using so-called '*non-screen*' film, involves an increased X-ray exposure but, because of the higher radiation dosage permitted to these areas, does not imply a significantly greater hazard to the patient.

(The use of 'non-screen' film has been discontinued in some X-ray departments because of difficulties with automatic processing.)

Foreign bodies. Demonstration of opaque foreign bodies or minute pathological opacities are techniques for which direct exposure of film is sometimes used to eliminate the possibility of screen artefacts.

Dental. Intra-oral dental radiographs (i.e., those exposed within the mouth) are usually taken without intensifying screens. Reasons include elimination of screen unsharpness and obviously, the awkwardness of placing a cassette in the patient's mouth.

Summary

Intensifying screens are used to minimise (1) risk of patient movement during exposures and (2) radiation hazards.

The type of screens will be chosen to satisfy particular circumstances:

— whether radiation protection is of prime importance (fast screens)
— or minimising risk of movement (fast screens)
— or where photographic unsharpness needs to be restricted (slower screens).

In all cases, screens must be clean and cassettes in good condition.

For some examinations, it may be preferred not to use intensifying screens.

Suggested exercises

Students should find out:

— How many types of intensifying screens (speeds, phosphors) are used in the X-ray department; for what examinations they are variously used; and if there are any possible exceptions to this practice.
— If there are different types of (ordinary) cassette in use in the department; if so why — and which seems most satisfactory.
— Whether there are also any specialised cassettes (curved, multisection).
— How cassettes are identified.
— How frequently the screens are cleaned — and by what method.
— What test is performed on cassettes suspected of having

poor screen/film contact. (This test should be carried out by students, under supervision.)
— Whether there are any other items of equipment, apart from cassettes, in the X-ray department which incorporate intensifying screens.

Related studies

Intensifying screen construction; types of screen; different phosphors; cleaning of screens. Cassette types: their construction and maintenance.

6

What happens to an X-ray film while it is being processed?

Exposure, alone, creates no visible change in the appearance of an X-ray film. The fact that some short of change *does* occur, however, is confirmed by processing: the uniformly yellow-green film is converted into a **radiograph**.

This transformation usually takes place out of sight inside an automatic processing machine. It involves two chemical stages — **development** and **fixation** — followed by **washing** with water and, finally, **drying**.

Development

It is during this stage that the changes produced by exposure are detected. In an unexposed emulsion, each silver halide crystal is surrounded by a barrier of negative ions. Breaks occur in the barriers around *exposed* crystals; these form an invisible pattern on the film, termed a **latent image**.

Photographic developing agents are chemicals, capable of distinguishing between exposed and unexposed crystals — a property termed '**selectivity**'. This is concerned with the developer's being a source, or 'donor', of electrons.

The intact, negative ion barriers around unexposed crystals tend to repel external electrons and therefore remain unaffected — i.e., undeveloped. The incomplete barriers around exposed crystals, however, allow electrons to penetrate. Their effect is to convert positive silver ions into neutral atoms; thus an *exposed* silver halide crystal is developed into a minute speck of metallic **silver**.

In this way, development *converts a latent image into a visible image*, with silver being created in the areas affected by, and in quantities proportional to, exposure. (This silver is finely-divided and black, and bears no resemblance to the more familiar, polished form.)

Reference has been made to the developing agent's selectivity: ideally this is a 100% discrimination. In practice, however, it is less than ideal: some *unexposed* crystals also are converted into silver. The extent to which this occurs, depends on development conditions: with careful control, it can be minimised.

'Developer' is a chemical solution in which films are immersed. In this way, the developer's chemicals are able to react with the film's (exposed) chemicals. If allowed to continue indefinitely, this reaction would result in conversion of *all* silver halide, whether exposed or not, into silver — i.e., there would be no image. Development is therefore allowed to proceed up to, but not beyond, a predetermined point. The time required depends on the developer solution's composition, concentration and temperature.

Fixation

Since development concerns the exposed crystals in a film emulsion, a developed film contains *unchanged* silver halide which is still *sensitive to light*. Thus not only must there be protection against light during development, but a developed image is not stable: it needs to be made *insensitive* to light. This process is termed **fixation**.

When removed from the developer solution, a film still retains in its emulsions an amount of the solution, which is *alkaline*. The fixer solution, however, is *acidic* and thus achieves its preliminary purpose — of terminating development — by *neutralisation*.

The fixing agent removes unexposed silver halide crystals from a film emulsion, leaving the silver image unaffected. Removal is achieved by conversion of the silver halide into a product which is soluble in water. This is then washed out of the emulsion.

Whereas development is a process which is terminated before its effects begin to reduce image quality, fixation has an obvious end-point — i.e., when all the remaining silver halide has been removed. The time allowed for a film to be fixed is thus not as critical as the time determined for its development.

Washing

At the end of fixation, a radiograph appears to have completed its processing: the silver image is seen against a clear background. But the 'clear' parts of the radiograph are, at this stage, *saturated* with *surplus fixer* and the *products of fixation*. If allowed to remain in the film, these chemicals will crystallise and decompose; eventually they stain and obscure image details.

Fixed radiographs therefore need to be **washed** thoroughly. Immersion in 'running' (rapidly-changing) water allows residual chemicals to diffuse out of the emulsions. Washing is allowed to continue until the chemical concentration in the emulsions has been reduced to a very low, safe level.

Drying

Lastly, excess water needs to be removed from the emulsions. As they leave the washing tank, films pass between 'squeegee' rollers which squeeze out a considerable amount of water. The remainder (down to the humidity of the atmosphere) is removed by *infra-red radiation* and jets of *warm air*.

Hardening

X-ray film emulsions need to be **hardened** — i.e., to be made *resistant to swelling* when wet. A swollen gelatin emulsion is susceptible to physical damage, especially when warm, during transport through a processor.

Hardening is not a single action but is sustained through the first stages of the processing cycle. Separate hardeners are included in the emulsion, in the developer solution and in the fixer, to restrict emulsion swelling.

Suggested exercises

A helpful way for students to observe the effects of processing chemicals on film emulsions is to process some films in dishes. Exposed films of phantoms or other test objects must be used for this purpose. Moderately weak solutions of developer and fixer should be used so that they will act only slowly.

Since this is an experimental exercise, it may be found useful to deviate from correct practices:

— The level of safelighting can be increased, to allow image changes to be observed more easily.
— The effects may be seen of
  a. switching on a white light as soon as the film is placed into fixer
  b. shortening and prolonging the development time
  c. omission of washing (simply allow a fixed film to dry off)
  d. processing at different temperatures.
N.B. Precautions must be taken to protect hands and clothing (gloves and an apron are recommended); and films may be handled with tongs.

Related studies

The chemical composition of processing solutions; formation of the latent image; consequences of errors in the processing cycle.

7

Why are radiographs usually processed in an automatic machine?

To appreciate the answer to this question, it will be helpful to look briefly at the history of processing. For the first 50 years, radiographs were processed *manually* — that is, the radiographer or darkroom technician moved films by hand through the stages of processing, using a clockwork timer to signal when a film was due to be moved on. The manual system gave general satisfaction but there could be problems:

— the 'setting' of the timing clock could be occasionally overlooked — and the final ring of its bell ignored.
— films were susceptible to damage — sometimes becoming detached from their hangers and sinking to the bottom of the tanks.
  (Both these faults could lead to repeat radiographs being required.)
— the departmental darkroom, although centrally sited, could require time-consuming journeys from the radiographic rooms on the outer margins of the department.
— the darkroom, with its open tanks of chemicals emitting fumes, could be an unpleasant working environment.

The first automation in film processing was introduced to *standardise* processing and eliminate handling marks. This was achieved simply by the devising of a transport system, driven by an electric motor. In parallel with this photographic innovation, X-ray exposure automation, so familiar today, was being introduced. The two were complementary: an automatic exposure timer being ineffective if processing standards fluctuated; an automatic processor being of reduced value if it simply perpetuated errors in exposure factor selection.

Designers of the early autoprocessors paid attention to achieving faultless and consistent processing, rather than shortening the time of the 'dry-to-dry' cycle. But in response to 'consumer demand' improvements were introduced to bring the cycle time below 10 minutes, then down to 7, $3\frac{1}{2}$ and finally $1\frac{1}{2}$ minutes. This achievement became possible through a remodelling of every component in the system; and, importantly, through a new emphasis on *accuracy*.

Manual processing had involved chemical solutions at 'room temperature' — usually 20°C. Typical development time was nominally 4 minutes; but variation of a few seconds more or less made no detectable difference to the radiographic images. Neither did a slight change in temperature, and the chemical concentrations of the solutions were also permitted to fluctuate.

Steps to reduce cycle time included *increasing operating temperatures* and, by new formulation, *raising the chemical activity* of processing solutions. These changes were not easily achieved. An increase above room temperature necessitated continuous and controlled heating; film construction had to be modified; and, as well as in their original formulation, an *accurate system of replenishing* the chemical solutions had to be devised.

The result of all these changes — as it were, the price which had to be paid for achieving a 90-second cycle — was that *every operating condition became critical*: there was no longer room for error. The need for greater accuracy was accompanied by an increased emphasis on cleanliness to reduce risks of contamination and damage.

A modern automatic film processor is a very reliable piece of equipment. Its main benefits are that:

1. Standardisation of processing complements the care taken in exposure factor selection;
2. The short processing cycle helps to minimise the time patients are kept waiting in the X-ray department;

3. Compact design has enabled processors to be distributed at convenient sites throughout a department.

But students must appreciate that the performance of an auto-processor cannot be taken for granted: it requires correct management and maintenance.

Suggested exercises

Students should
— Closely inspect an automatic processing machine — inside and out!
— Ask members of staff responsible for the machine, about:

   a. how chemical solutions are mixed
   b. the system of accurately replenishing the solutions
   c. checks on temperatures, water flow, and electrical supply
   d. correct film feeding procedure
   e. cleaning and safety.

— Find out, in simple terms, how the day-to-day consistency of a machine's performance is monitored; and how it is accurately matched to other autoprocessors within the X-ray department.

Related studies

Processing chemical formulation and replenishment, and aspects of film construction relevant to automatic systems of processing; the construction, operation and maintenance of an autoprocessor.

8

Why does a darkroom have lights?

It can come as a surprise to a new student to find that X-ray darkrooms are illuminated, rather than being places of total blackness. Apart from the 'white' lights used at times when films are not being processed, there are also **safelights** to which a film may be exposed without being '**fogged**' — i.e. without *unintentional* densities being added to its image.

Safelighting is feasible due to the fact that X-ray film's colour sensitivity is mainly restricted to a *specific range of wavelengths*. The range is chosen to coincide with emissions from the intensifying screens used with the film. It follows that X-ray film has a *limited sensitivity to other wavelengths* in the visible spectrum. These are therefore available for use as safelighting — usually red/brown light, since X-ray films are sensitive to blue or blue/green.

It must be understood that such 'safety' *is not absolute*: although X-ray film's greatest sensitivity is to other wavelengths, it is to some extent sensitive to those transmitted by the safelights. If left for long enough in this light, a film will become fogged. A further point, although simple, might be mentioned: the restricted colour sensitivity of an X-ray film emulsion affords no safety from exposure to 'white' light, since this comprises *all* wavelengths.

When darkroom illumination is planned, consideration is

33

given to safelight **intensity** as well as colour. Planning takes two interests into account. On the one hand, there is a case for keeping safelighting as *dim* as possible to minimise the hazards to *image quality*. On the other hand, *bright* illumination provides the *least unpleasant* working conditions for darkrooms personnel, and *lessens the risk of accidents* when handling chemicals and equipment. The eventual intensity is a compromise between these two conflicting requirements.

A criterion termed the '**safe handling time**' is applied to safelighting intensity. This is a reasonably generous assessment of the time needed to take a film through all the stages between its initial removal from the film hopper and eventual insertion into the autoprocessor. It should be possible for a film (of the fastest type, if different speeds are in use) to be exposed to a darkroom's safelights for 30–40 seconds *without acquiring any extra detectable fog*.

The required intensity is provided by an appropriate number of safelights (considering the size of the room) assisted by light-coloured, softly-reflecting paint on the ceiling and walls.

Conventional safelights take the form of lantern-like, metal boxes fitted with coloured glass filters allowing light of only the required wavelength range to be transmitted. There are two types:(i) the *direct* safelight which has a filter forming its under side, to cast light down onto the bench surface; (ii) the type, usually ceiling-suspended above the floor area, incorporating *two filters* — one below and one above. These provide both downward, direct light and indirect upward light which reflects from the ceiling to give diffused, general illumination.

The light source inside safelights is usually a *25-watt* electric lamp. The relatively low heat output suits the fact that the safelight housing has to prevent the escape of unfiltered, white light — i.e., there are no ventilation holes.

Students will also note that a darkroom has all its entrances (doors and cassette hatches) lightproofed to protect films against exposure to 'white' light.

Suggested exercises

— At a convenient time, when film processing is not in

progress, students should inspect an example of each type
of safelight used in the X-ray department's darkrooms.
— A simple experiment can be performed to assess the 'safe'
length of time for which a film may be left lying on the
darkroom bench. This involves using a mask which is
retracted across the film to create a series of parallel areas,
each exposed for a different time. An unexposed strip is
left to act as a 'control'. The test should be carried out
according to the X-ray department's practice.

Related studies

Spectral sensitivity of X-ray film emulsions; construction of the
various types of safelights and filters; general methods of
providing and testing safelight illumination; maintenance of
safelights.

9

Is a darkroom always necessary?

The purpose of a conventional X-ray darkroom includes protection of films against exposure to white light, when they are:

— unpacked from (manufacturers') boxes
— placed in the hopper
— loaded into cassettes
— unloaded from cassettes
— identified with patients' data
— inserted into an autoprocessor.

For many years, the benefits which automatic processing brought to an X-ray department were accepted as sufficient. The continued search for efficiency, however, turned people's attention to the fact that the old darkroom techniques before the processing stage, could also be modernised.

An early improvement was the introduction of so-called 'daylight' identification systems. These enabled a film to be marked with the patient's details, while still in the cassette. But the procedures of loading and unloading cassettes could also be mechanised. So, to replace the darkroom film hopper a *dispensing machine* for loading film into cassettes was introduced; and an *unloading device* was added to the feed-in section of an autoprocessor. These innovations meant that procedures which previously required safelighting could now be performed safely *outside* a darkroom.

There are now in use, two main types of **'daylight' processing system**. One requires the operator to perform the *two separate stages* of cassette loading and unloading, with several film dispensers (for different sizes) dispersed around a processor. The other has a single, centralised unit which automatically performs *all* the stages, without assistance. There are also processors fitted 'end-on' to X-ray equipment which is virtually *'cassette-less'*, having automated film handling throughout a radiographic technique.

Thus a darkroom is *not* always necessary. Benefits to an X-ray department of having a 'daylight' system are both *photographic* — eliminating the risks both of safelight fog and handling artefacts — and *time-saving*, so that work can be streamlined.

But the introduction of a daylight system into an existing department is expensive: structural alterations are needed as well as the capital outlay on equipment. The design of some older X-ray departments may in fact preclude or, at least, fail to justify the cost of a changeover. It may be found that, even with a daylight system, the X-ray department needs to retain a darkroom or safelit loading room, for the film magazines of rapid changers and cameras, as well as for multi-section and other special cassettes.

Suggested exercises

— Students who have the opportunity, in the course of their practical work, to see both daylight and conventional systems in operation, should compare the two, in their separate contexts.

— A comparison exercise, involving efficiency, can be undertaken by students having the opportunity to experience use of two different daylight systems.

— Students with no current experience of daylight processing could try to discover what plans there might be for a changeover — or why such a move might have been discounted.

Related studies

Daylight processing systems: construction and operation; advantages and limitations.

10

Can radiographic images be misleading?

Radiographic images can suffer from excess unsharpness and lack of contrast. These faults reduce diagnostic value and are potentially misleading, but they can be corrected by careful radiographic technique. There is another problem, however, which is both permanent and unavoidable: a radiograph only shows two dimensions. An object's 'length' and 'width' are demonstrated but its 'depth' — i.e., the dimension *along the axis of the X-ray beam* — is not recorded.

To a limited extent, comparisons can be made between radiographs and photographs. A photograph is also two-dimensional — whether printed on paper or projected on to a screen. But a photographer can employ techniques not available to a radiographer: the 'depth' of a photographic subject can be portrayed or, at least, suggested by perspective, and light and shade.

A reasonable comparison might also be made with the illusion a children's entertainer can create, by projecting silhouettes of hands and fingers on to a screen to resemble birds and animals. The illusionist turns to advantage the conditions which make a radiographer's task difficult: that shadows cast, one upon another, can obscure and deceive.

When analysed, the restriction of a radiographic image to two dimensions raises problems of **distortion** and **superimposition**.

39

Distortion

This may be defined as *alteration in shape* — that is, when the image does not correspond to the shape of the object. It can arise from either or both of two separate causes.

Elongation

Radiographic images are *larger than the objects they repre-sent*. This is due to divergence of the X-ray beam and separation between object and image planes (Fig. 9). The **magnification factor** — that is, the relationship between image and object sizes — is the *ratio* of distances between (i) *focal spot (source of X-rays) and film* and (ii) *focal spot and object*.

Unless precise measurement of the object is required (or if the image is enlarged beyond the size of the film!) magnification is not a significant problem, provided that it is *equal*, across the whole of the object. This condition is satisfied by having the *object plane parallel to the film*.

If magnification is not equal across the object — i.e., if it does not lie parallel to the film — *elongation* will occur, as shown in Figure 10.

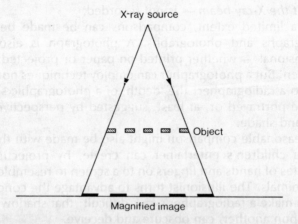

Fig. 9 An object at 90° to the central X-ray and parallel to the film, produces a magnified image. In this case the equal spacing between adjacent alternating areas is preserved.

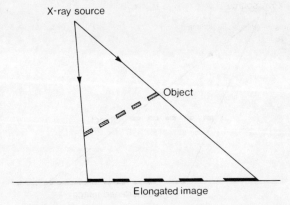

Fig. 10 Angulation of an object, in relation to the film, causes image elongation. In this case, there is an increasing magnification of adjacent areas.

Foreshortening

For every object, there is a generally agreed conception of its shape. A solid, three-dimensional object can be viewed from many angles, but there are likely to be certain views of it which are considered 'best' — i.e., most recognisable and informative. For example: if several anatomy textbooks are consulted, it is likely that their illustrations of the various organs and other three-dimensional structures within the body will be found to be very similar.

Standard radiographic views, or **projections**, are based on the same principle. If, however, the X-ray beam does *not* approach an object along the required line of view, there will be an oblique distortion, due to lack of the third dimension, known as *foreshortening* (Fig. 11). Radiographic positioning should therefore provide for the *object plane to lie at right angles to the X-ray beam*.

Foreshortening and elongation

Students must appreciate that these two forms of distortion occur *independently*:

Foreshortening is associated with the angle at which the X-ray beam from the tube, approaches the object.

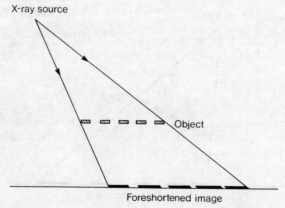

Fig. 11 An oblique approach by the X-ray beam foreshortens the image: the equal proportion between adjacent, alternating areas, is lost.

Elongation can occur when the transmitted X-ray beam, carrying the shadows of the object, meets the film.

Thus, both forms of distortion can occur *simultaneously*, as illustrated in Figure 12. It should be noted that foreshortening and elongation are *not* direct opposites: an increase in one *cannot* compensate for an excess of the other. Careful radiographic technique will minimise both.

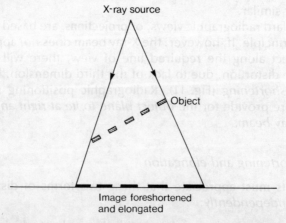

Fig. 12 Oblique approach by the X-ray beam and unequal magnification cause complex distortion.

Superimposition

This hazard of image production is relatively easy to understand. Since a radiograph is formed by the passage of an X-ray beam *through* an object, it follows that every structure lying in the path of the beam may cast a shadow. A radiographic image is thus a composite of many shadows.

Structures aligned together in the path of the beam cast shadows which **superimpose**, one upon another, with the *densest tending to be dominant*. In this way, the less dense structures can be obliterated altogether or have misleading patterns superimposed on them by other structures. Again, careful radiographic technique minimises this occurrence.

Suggested exercise

— With guidance from an experienced radiographer, students should examine some radiographs for examples of distortion and superimposition.

Related studies

The geometry of image formation.

11

How do radiographers assess the technical quality of their radiographs?

Before exposing a radiograph, there are a number of steps to be taken to make the image as informative as possible. Radiographers are required to make a careful choice of equipment and accessories, and to be precise in positioning the patient, the film and the X-ray tube.

When processed and ready for viewing, every radiograph should confirm the following points:

The whole of the required anatomical area is shown

The extent of this will be determined by circumstances: it must be ensured that all areas of potential value to a full diagnosis are included; but there will also be a tendency for the field to be minimised in order to limit harmful radiation radiation effects.

The object is, if required, shown in a particular functional state

This could be as simple as the arrested inspiration required of a patient during radiography of the chest, or need to be as precisely timed (synchronised) as a particular phase during a blood-flow study.

The image is virtually free from distortion and superimposed shadows

Accepted criteria are laid down for assessing this aspect of most radiographic projections. Because of the two-dimensional limitations of a single radiograph, two or more views may need to be considered together to satisfy this requirement completely.

There is only a minimal amount of unsharpness

Being aware of all the possible causes of unsharpness, the radiographer will have attempted to equalise these, down to the lowest level achievable in the circumstances.

The image has the required density and contrast

Involved here are accurate estimation of the 'size' of the object, careful use of equipment and selection of exposure factors.

There are no artefacts or other photographic blemishes

Some of these are beyond anticipation but many can be avoided by careful preparation and technique.

All necessary identification data must be clearly shown

Of all these points, this is probably the easiest to achieve.

A final point must be added, concerning *radiation protection of the patient*: the above technical criteria must be met, using the smallest practicable X-ray exposure. Confirmation that this has been so, might not be obvious from the radiographic appearances, but the radiographer concerned must be satisfied that appropriate precautions have been taken.

Suggested exercise

— Students should observe how experienced radiographers go through this exercise with a range of radiographs.

12

How many factors influence radiographic image contrast?

The **contrast** of a radiograph is an expression of the *difference between photographic densities*. The term may be applied either to the *whole* of a radiograph to express the recorded range of densities, from highest to lowest; or to a *single structure*, as a measure of the density difference between its particular image and the immediate surroundings (see Fig. 13). In whichever sense the term is used, there are many influences on the eventual image from which diagnosis is made. These will be described in the sequence summarised in Figure 14.

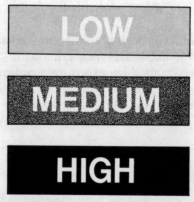

Fig. 13 Degrees of image contrast.

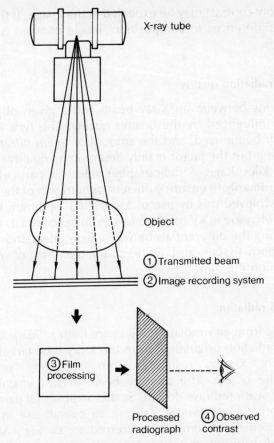

Fig. 14 Radiographic image contrast: four stages of influence.

TRANSMITTED BEAM

The pattern of radiation intensities within the X-ray beam emerging from an object may be thought of as the 'raw material' upon which subsequent stages of image production exert their effects. It is principally influenced by:

Composition of the object

The various structures within the object, of differing *density*, *effective atomic number* and *thickness*, determine whether high or low contrast may be expected in the image. If there are marked differences in composition, image contrast is potentially high.

Incident radiation quality

Interactions between an X-ray beam and a given object are strongly influenced by the beam's **quality**. The *type of X-ray generator* being used, and the amount of *beam filtration* can influence it but the factor mainly determining quality is the **X-ray tube kilovoltage**. A radiographer selects a particular kilovoltage primarily to ensure sufficient *penetration* of the object. Having achieved this by use of a so-called 'optimum kilovoltage', an *increase* in kV tends to *lessen* image contrast, through (i) reducing the differentials between X-ray attenuation by the various body tissues, and (ii) increasing the effect of scattered radiation on the film.

Scattered radiation

Emerging from an irradiated object are both *primary* X-rays — that is, radiation originating from the X-ray tube target — and *secondary* X-rays, resulting from scattering processes within the object. The primary beam carries image 'information'; scattered rays do not. Scatter exposes all parts of the film, more or less evenly, causing an overall rise in photographic densities, commonly referred to as '**fog**'. Although equally distributed, this added density is *more noticeable in the lower density areas of the image*. Thus its effect is to *reduce contrast*.

The radiographer has some control, however, over both the amount of scattered radiation *produced* and, of this, the proportion which *reaches the X-ray film*.

Restriction of scatter production

One simple method of restricting the amount of scatter produced, is by *limiting the X-ray field size*. In this way, the volume of tissue exposed to the primary beam, is reduced (see Fig. 15).

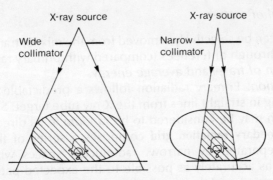

Fig. 15 Reduction in amount of scattered radiation produced: primary beam collimation lessens the volume of tissue irradiated.

If an abdominal structure is being radiographed, a further technique can be employed to reduce the volume of tissue irradiated, particularly if the patient is obese. This technique is usually termed '**compression**' (see Fig. 16). The term may be considered misleading, however, since — although patients feel they are being compressed — the action is really one of tissue *displacement*. In addition to restricting the volume of scatter-producing tissue, there are two other benefits: *immobilisation* is assisted and, because the abdomen is temporarily made 'thinner', the *required X-ray exposure is reduced*.

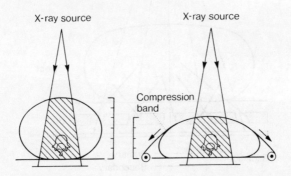

Fig. 16 Reduction in amount of scattered radiation produced: abdominal compression (displacement) reduces the volume of tissue irradiated by the primary beam. Note also the reduced object dimension (thickness) required to be penetrated by the X-ray beam.

Removal of scatter

Scatter can be selectively removed from the mixed, transmitted beam, through differences (compared with primary rays) in its *direction of travel* and *average energy*.

Direction. Primary radiation follows a predictable path — diverging in straight lines from the X-ray tube target. Scattered radiation may be considered to be *random* in its direction.

A **secondary radiation grid** comprises a series of thin lead strips separated by narrow, radiolucent spaces which are aligned as accurately as possible to the expected path of the X-ray beam. A grid thus freely allows passage of image-forming radiation but presents absorbing barriers to the scatter which is not travelling along these permitted paths (see Fig. 17).

Increasing separation between object and film improves the likelihood that obliquely-travelling scatter will 'miss' the film, while primary continues directly towards the film. This forms

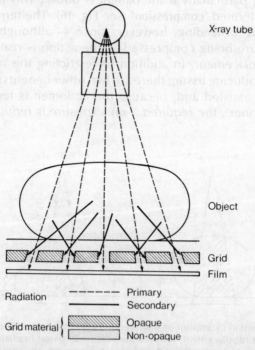

X-ray tube

Object

Grid

Film

Radiation		
	- - - - -	Primary
	———	Secondary

Grid material
Opaque
Non-opaque

Fig. 17 Reduction in the amount of scatter (secondary radiation) reaching the film. Cross section through grid (diagrammatic) to show its selective action.

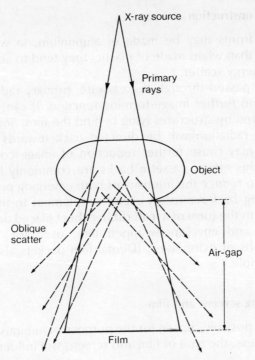

Fig. 18 Reduction in the amount of scatter (secondary radiation) reaching the film. Principle of an air gap.

the principle of an '**air gap**' (see Fig. 18). An air gap is not without its drawbacks, however. It increases the risk of image unsharpness and is much less practicable than the use of a grid. It is most often seen used as a consequential feature of the image enlargement technique, *macroradiography*.

Average energy. Scattered radiation is less energetic than primary radiation: thus it is more easily attenuated. By simply positioning a thin metal sheet (tin or aluminium) between object and film, scatter is preferentially **filtered** out of the beam.

IMAGE RECORDING SYSTEM

This comprises film and intensifying screens and, usually, a cassette.

Cassette construction

Cassette fronts may be made of aluminium, in which case (more so than when made of plastic) they tend to act as *filters* of low-energy scatter.

Having passed through the cassette, primary radiation can perform no further image-forming function. It can, however, be scattered by structures lying behind the film. Some of this scattered radiation will be directed back towards the film, where it may cause further reduction of image contrast. To counter this effect, cassette backs are commonly lined with lead foil to reduce the intensity of both emerging primary and re-entering *back-scatter*. A useful supplement to this can be provided in the form of a lead rubber sheet placed underneath cassettes and envelope-wrapped film, used for 'table-top' radiographs of extremities. (Dental film packets also employ this principle.)

Intensifying screens and film

Although possibly chosen for the purpose of minimising image unsharpness, the type of film and screens will influence image contrast.

Intensifying screens

The intensifying process, by which X-rays are converted into longer-wavelength light and ultraviolet radiation, becomes more efficient as X-ray energy increases — although the nature of this change depends on the type of phosphor in the screen. For this reason, longer-wavelength scattered radiation has *less effect* on the image, and contrast is improved.

Film

Film emulsions have individual *sensitometric* characteristics. These variations, in response to exposure whether by X-rays or screen emissions, form an interesting and important subject for students' attention. For present purposes, however, it is sufficient to note that image contrast is one of an emulsion's most important features.

The age of a film — in terms of its 'freshness' — is also

significant: films acquire '*storage fog*' if stored in unsuitable conditions or for too long before use.

FILM PROCESSING

Safelighting

Both before and after exposure, a film may need to be handled under darkroom safelighting conditions. If these provide the correct wavelength and intensity, the film will undergo no changes. But if darkroom illumination is *not* 'safe' or if a film is exposed for *longer* than the allowed 'handling time', *safelight fog* will occur, reducing image contrast.

Development

Development is the stage of processing during which invisible, latent images become visible. Ideally, a developing agent will act only on *exposed* areas of film emulsion, creating densities in proportion to the quantities of absorbed radiation energy. In practice, this ideal is not achieved: some development of unexposed silver halide occurs to produce '*chemical*' or '*development*' *fog*. The extent to which this reduces contrast, can be controlled — influential factors including chemical formulation and concentration, development time and temperature. (Again, this is a complex subject, requiring close attention from students, at a later stage).

VIEWING CONDITIONS

When a radiograph is viewed, the only light seen should be that transmitted through the radiograph. Light from other sources will have the effect of reducing the '*subjective*' contrast appreciated by the person viewing the radiograph.

Transmitted light

The contrast within a finished radiographic image can be seen fully, only if a correctly illuminated viewing screen is used.

Light intensity must be equal across the whole screen area, and should be adjustable to match the average density of any given radiograph so that its contrast is seen to best advantage.

Extraneous light

Direct light, shining from the viewing screen around a radiograph's borders, can dazzle a person viewing the image. Viewing screens should be fitted with *adjustable shutters* to mask off such extraneous light.

Reflected light

Room lighting reflected from a radiograph's surface is seen, adding to the transmitted light emerging from the image. Although this additional light might be even across the film's surface, it will be *most noticeable in the high density (darker) areas* and virtually unnoticeable in the areas of low density. Its effect is thus to reduce subjective appreciation of contrast, by shortening the range of light intensities.

Summary

A dozen or so of the possible influences on image contrast have been outlined. There are others, however, and gaining a full understanding of image contrast will probably occupy a student's attention for much of the training course. The simple four-stage description given, has been offered as the simplest introduction to the various causes, but students may be further helped by an alternative analysis which considers the factors in two groups: those which (i) concern *demonstration of the object*, and (ii) only add *background density* to the image.

Included in the first group are *tube kilovoltage, film/screen characteristics* and, naturally, *object composition*. The second group includes *scattered radiation, fog* (from film storage, safelighting and processing) and *viewing conditions*.

Suggested exercises

— Under the supervision of an experienced radiographer,

students should look at a collection of radiographs, to assess and comment on image contrast. In cases where there is low contrast, it should be determined whether this is due to composition of the object, deliberate adjustment by the radiographer, or the combined effects of 'fogging' factors.

— Some radiographs should be viewed under (i) ideal and (ii) unsuitable conditions; the effects on subjective contrast should be noted.

— With the use of an anatomical phantom, a series of test radiographs should be produced, showing the effects upon contrast of: kV adjustment, use of a secondary radiation grid, primary beam collimation and different film/screen combinations. (Some of these effects can be conveniently demonstrated by fluoroscopy, if suitable equipment is available.)

Related studies

The interactions of X-rays with matter; influences on X-ray beam quality; film emulsion characteristics; composition of developing solutions; development conditions and their effects.

13

What might cause a radiographic image to be unsharp?

Radiographic image unsharpness may be due to any of a number of causes. These are usually classified as:

— belonging to a group of **geometric** factors
— associated with **movement** during the exposure
— being **photographic** in origin.

When a patient is radiographed, these various causes usually bear some relationship to one another, and the radiographer's skill is needed to achieve a balance between them. For these introductory purposes, however, three separate descriptions are given.

Geometric unsharpness

The reason why *un*sharpness is discussed, rather than sharpness, is that every radiographic image — however perfect in other respects — is considered to have some degree of unsharpness. One permanent cause of this is to be found within the X-ray tube. Here, the source of the X-rays — the **focal spot**, or **focus** — *is not a point source*. If it were, (see Fig. 19a) reduction of unsharpness would be a much simpler task for the radiographer.

Whereas visible light can be focused by lenses and mirrors

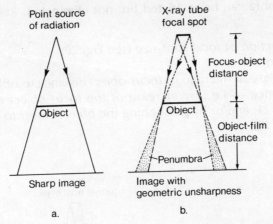

Fig. 19 Radiographic image formation with (a) an ideal (theoretical) radiation source, and (b) a practical source.

to behave as if originating from a point source, X-rays have to be used 'as they come' from the focal spot. Although very small, the focal spot behaves as *a group* of point sources instead of as a single point source. In Figure 19b, the point sources at the extreme edges of the focal spot are considered. Each casts a separate shadow of the object. Although these fall very close together, *they do not exactly coincide*: thus around the edge of the complete shadow is a zone of *incomplete* shadow, termed **penumbra**. Penumbra is not homogeneous: it becomes more marked from its outside edge, in towards the central, full shadow. This gives a blurred appearance to the edges of every object's shadow within a radiographic image, termed *geometric unsharpness*.

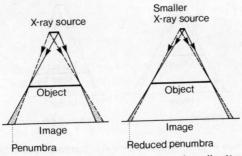

Fig. 20 Reduction in geometric unsharpness: use of smaller X-ray source.

Penumbra can be restricted but not eliminated. Restriction requires

— *reduction of focal spot size* (see Fig. 20)
  and/or
— increase of the ratio of *focus-object* distance to *object-film* distance — i.e., by *increase of the focus-object distance* (Fig. 21) and/or by positioning the *object closer to the film* (Fig. 22).

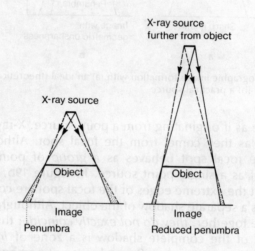

Fig. 21 Reduction in geometric unsharpness: increase of ratio between focus-object distance and object-film distance. (Compare with Fig. 22.)

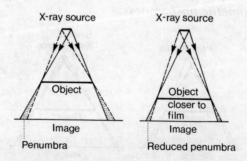

Fig. 22 Reduction in geometric unsharpness: increase of ratio between focus-object distance and object-film distance. (Compare with Fig. 21.)

Movement (kinetic) unsharpness

If an object moves during the exposure, its image will be blurred. Movement unsharpness may be prevented if a radiographer successfully pays attention to:

— immobilising the object
— minimising the exposure time.

Immobilisation

(a) Clear communication is important between radiographer and patient. During some X-ray examinations — although quite routine, as far as the radiographer is concerned — patients can be genuinely surprised to hear that they are expected to hold their breath for the duration of an exposure! Every patient should be given a full *explanation* of a procedure, before it begins; and if a breathing manoeuvre is involved, a *rehearsal* will be valuable.
(b) Patients' *comfort* is important: a comfortable patient feels more restful and less inclined to move.
(c) Various devices are available to help keep an object still during exposures: foam plastic pads (within the beam) and sandbags or other weights (outside the beam) for example.

Exposure time

Exposure time is one of the two factors determining the quantity of radiation to which an X-ray film is exposed. **Radiation intensity** is the other factor (*quantity = intensity × time*). It is clear, therefore, that exposure time alone cannot be reduced for the purpose of eliminating movement unsharpness, unless a compensatory increase in radiation intensity is made. Otherwise, a film will be inadequately exposed.

Some of the factors under the radiographer's control, which influence radiation intensity — tube kilovoltage and focus-film distance, for example — exert other effects on the radiographic image (and are usually chosen for these other purposes), but **X-ray tube current** directly and without complication controls radiation intensity.

The *product* of tube current (measured in milliamperes) and exposure time (in seconds) is the quantity of electric charge which flows through the X-ray tube during an exposure, in *millicoulombs*. The unit **milliampere-second** (*mAs*) is customarily used to measure charge, in radiography, however. It is precisely the same as a millicoulomb but is perhaps more obviously the product of *mA* and *s*. Milliampere-seconds are used by radiographers to express, in an indirect but very practical way, the **quantity of radiation** produced in the X-ray tube. Thus, a certain mAs value will be specified to indicate the X-ray exposure needed for a given radiograph.

In order to minimise movement unsharpness, an mAs value will normally be the product of a *high tube current* and a *short exposure time*. For example, 60 mAs will be achieved by 500 mA × 0.12 s rather than by 100 mA × 0.6 s.

Photographic unsharpness

Unsharpness can be introduced into a radiographic image, at the stage where the radiation pattern transmitted through the patient acts on the *image recording system*.

Both the silver halide in a film emulsion and the phosphor in an intensifying screen are present in the form of crystals. These are very small and unlikely, in themselves, to be larger than the fine details of the object which need to be recorded on the image. The fluorescent emission from crystals in an intensifying screen is divergent, however, and *spreads its effect* over a larger area. An amount of reflection and energy scattering also occurs within screen and film emulsion. These effects (see Fig. 23) combine to introduce some *diffusion* into the radiation pattern, as recorded on the film.

Photographic unsharpness will be minimal when screens are used which have a *thin fluorescent layer* and incorporate some form of *pigment* to minimise the scattering and reflection of light.

It should be mentioned that poor screen/film contact increases the extent to which the emission from a screen crystal diverges before it reaches the film emulsion. In this way, the *condition of a cassette* affects photographic unsharpness.

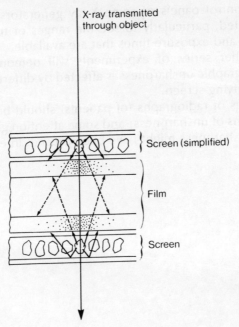

Fig. 23 Response of intensifying screens to an X-ray exposure. Light divergence and scattering increase the affected areas of the film emulsions.

Suggested exercises

— Penumbra can be seen surrounding the shadows of everyday objects in the path of visible light from the sun or from an electric lamp. A little experimentation will verify this effect.

— The components of a dismantled X-ray tube should be examined. The area on the anode where X-rays are produced should be viewed from the aspect it presents to an object being radiographed.

— A series of experiments to verify the influences upon geometric unsharpness should be planned and carried out, using an X-ray tube with two focal spots of different sizes, and an object such as a dry bone or a fine wire gauze.

— The control panels of some X-ray generators should be inspected, particularly to see the ranges of tube current values and exposure times that are available.
— A further series of experiments will demonstrate how photographic unsharpness is affected by different types of intensifying screen.
— A series of radiographs (of patients) should be inspected for signs of unsharpness; and some attention given to why the unsharpness might have been caused, in each case.

14

Why are radiographic projections standardised?

The answer to this question lies in the need to gain maximum diagnostic information about the patient, while creating the minimum radiation hazard.

Without standardisation, radiographic images would be diagnostically unreliable. If patients were positioned at random, somewhere between X-ray tube and film, their radiographs would tend to suffer from distortion, superimposition and excess unsharpness.

Instead, radiographers follow carefully planned procedures when positioning their patients, so that radiographs conform to a *recognised standard*.

It is important that these procedures can be *repeated identically*, with either the same patient or a succession of different patients to produce directly *comparable* images. In principle, therefore, the procedures are usually quite straightforward. They involve three aspects:

Positioning of the patient

The easiest positions for patients to adopt and consistently repeat are: supine, prone, and erect or seated, facing directly towards either the X-ray tube or the film. Intermediate lateral and oblique positions are also used.

Direction and centring of the X-ray beam

The beam is invariably centred to the middle of the object and is usually directed at right angles to the film. There are other circumstances, however, where the beam can be set at a measured angle other than 90° to approach the patient and the film obliquely.

Positioning of the film

The film is normally either horizontal or vertical and, since the X-ray beam is directed to the middle of the object, the film is usually also centred to the beam.

SOME STANDARD PROJECTIONS

Anteroposterior (commonly abbreviated to 'AP')

An anteroposterior projection is produced when the X-ray beam passes through the patient '*from the front to the back*'. The patient, or the anterior surface of the object, directly faces the X-ray tube, and the central ray of the beam passes along a sagittal plane.

Example
Anteroposterior projection of the thoracic spine
The patient lies supine on a horizontal X-ray couch, with the median plane centred and at right angles to the couch top.
The X-ray beam is vertical and centred in the midline to a point midway between the cricoid cartilage and the xiphoid process of the sternum (— through the sixth thoracic vertebra).
The film is placed in the bucky cassette tray and centred to the same point.

The median plane is fairly easily discerned, since the head, neck and trunk are symmetrical. Sagittal planes which pass through the limbs, however, are less obvious. When the limbs are radiographed, therefore, individual, *palpable bony landmarks* rather than standard planes, are used as positioning reference points.

Examples

For an AP projection of the ankle joint, the lateral and medial malleoli are positioned equidistant from the film; for an AP projection of the knee joint, the leg is adjusted by rotation, until the patella is centralised over the femur.

Postero-anterior (commonly abbreviated to 'PA')

Postero-anterior projections also involve direction of the X-ray beam along a sagittal plane, but in these cases the beam passes *'from the back to the front'*. The patient is positioned with the anterior surface of the body (or the part being examined) facing the film.

Example

Postero-anterior projection of the right hand

The patient is seated alongside the X-ray couch, with the right side nearer the couch. The right hand and forearm are pronated. The hand is placed in contact with and central to a film placed on the couch top. The fingers are extended and slightly separated. The vertical X-ray beam is centred to the dorsum at the head of the third metacarpal.

AP or PA?

Anteroposterior and postero-anterior projections have similarities: in both, the central X-ray passes along a sagittal plane; and both show the same dimensions of the object. When the object is relatively 'deep', however, some comparability will be lost due to the divergence of the oblique X-rays. Differences may be detectable in magnification, between anterior and posterior parts; or the beam's geometry may alter (by distortion) the shadows of certain parts of the object. These differences may be determining factors in the choice of whether to take AP or PA projections. Other possible factors include:

Anatomical considerations. An anteroposterior projection of the forearm is taken instead of a postero-anterior, because the radius crosses over the ulna when the hand is pronated. The shape of the ankle and foot would make a postero-anterior projection of the ankle a very awkward alternative to the anteroposterior.

The patient's comfort. The anteroposterior is a routine projection of the elbow joint; even a 'fit' patient would find difficulty or discomfort in being positioned for a postero-anterior projection.

Choice between AP or PA can be determined by the patient's injuries or illness: a fractured clavicle may be examined more comfortably by an anteroposterior projection than a PA; the bedridden patient usually has an anteroposterior projection of the chest, instead of the 'routine' PA.

Immobilisation. There would be no extra discomfort to the patient if anteroposterior projections of the hand and wrist were routine instead of postero-anterior. Pronation of the hand gives better stability of position, however — and is preferred by the patient. (Immobilisation and comfort are closely related.)

3. Lateral

A lateral (side) projection is the usual complement to an AP or PA; the X-ray beam travels along a coronal plane, to reveal the dimension of the object which is concealed on the AP and PA projections.

For lateral projections of the head, neck and trunk, the median plane is positioned parallel to the film.

> **Example**
> *Right lateral projection of the chest*
> The patient stands with the right side of the chest in contact with a vertical film. The patient's arms are raised and supported above the shoulders, and the position of the body is adjusted to bring the median plane parallel to the film.
> The horizontal X-ray beam is centred to the left axilla.

On lateral radiographs of the head, neck or trunk, *both halves* of the body, right and left, are shown *superimposed* upon each other. Through having less geometric unsharpness, however, the side nearer the film tends to be demonstrated more clearly.

Lateral projections of the limbs do not present the same problems of superimposition, since only one side (either right or left) is being examined. It is normally of little importance whether the lateral or the medial part of a limb should be shown more clearly than the other: accordingly, the choice of positioning, in this respect, is determined by the need for the patient to be comfortable. Thus, lateral projections of the wrist, forearm and elbow are taken with the medial side of the arm in contact with the film, while laterals of the knee joint and ankle joint are usually taken with the lateral aspect of the leg nearer the film.

The previously mentioned uncertainty of sagittal planes through the limbs is once more overcome by the use of bony landmarks so that lateral projections are actually taken at 90° to the AP and PA projections.

Inferosuperior and supero-inferior

These projections involve directing the X-ray beam vertically through the object — i.e., at right angles to a transverse body plane. They are employed as complements to AP, PA, or lateral projections, in circumstances determined by the shape and location of the object.

Examples

Whereas a lateral projection of the shoulder joint, in the conventional sense, would be of little diagnostic value (right and left sides being superimposed), an infero-superior projection may usefully complement the antero-posterior. The film is placed superiorly, in contact with the shoulder (arm abducted) and the X-ray beam is directed at 90° towards it, through the axilla.

A supero-inferior projection may be taken of the nasal bones, to complement a lateral projection, since neither an AP nor a PA will show the nasal bones through the dense superimposed shadows of the cranium.

Other projections

The types of projection described so far, bear a strictly perpendicular relationship to the planes of the body. It is as if they are 'surveys' of the body, from the principal 'points of the compass'. One reason for this simplicity has already been mentioned: the need for easily reproduced, comparable radiographs. But it may have struck the reader that these projections correspond to many of the conventional diagrams — aspects and sections — with which anatomy books are illustrated. This is not merely a coincidence; the correlation between radiographic projections and their counterpart anatomical illustrations is an aid to interpretation. But whereas the artist's skill with his pen can convey perspective on a diagram, a radiographic image can suffer from defects — some natural shapes being distorted and structures obscured by superimposition.

It would be unreasonable to expect that all the organs and other structures within the body, are so shaped and aligned as to be displayed on AP, PA, lateral and supero-inferior or inferosuperior projections, without distortion or superimposition. Not surprisingly, therefore, these projections may be found to have such defects. They serve their purposes as 'surveys' excellently, however: the slight distortion with which some structures are represented does not rob the projections of their diagnostic value. Three factors account for this: the anatomical knowledge of the person interpreting the radiograph; this person's experience of having seen numerous identical images before, and having been trained to interpret them; and the quality of the given radiograph — particularly in terms of its correct positioning.

This last point deserves important consideration by the student radiographer. An image produced by *symmetrical positioning* of the object and *precise centring* of the X-ray beam will present what may be termed 'acceptable distortion' — because it is expected and unavoidable. Thus, a symmetrical postero-anterior chest or anteroposterior abdomen will show some distortion which is familiar to a trained observer and can be taken into account when a diagnosis is made. Problems arise when the projection is *not* correct — i.e., when the patient has been allowed to *rotate* away from the required symmetrical position, and/or when the direction and centring of the X-ray beam have been *inaccurate*.

Nevertheless, it is the case — even with perfectly symmetrical AP, PA, lateral and supero-inferior or inferosuperior projections — that some structures are very distorted or completely obscured by superimposition. Clearer demonstration is possible with *oblique* projections or *tangential* projections designed to overcome these defects.

Suggested exercises

— Students should examine a series of radiographs, identify the radiographic projections and, with help from a radiographer, assess whether they are accurate.
— AP and PA radiographs of (i) the chest, and (ii) the abdomen should be compared for signs of how the X-ray beam geometry has affected appearances.

Related studies

Students will progressively learn the projections and techniques for radiographing the various parts of the body. Attention should be given to the criteria for checking the symmetry and accuracy of each projection.

Surface anatomy and experience in palpating skeletal landmarks should accompany learning of radiographic techniques.

15

How do standard projections enable superimposition to be minimised?

The problem of superimposition — i.e. of a structure's being obscured by the shadows of another, more radiopaque structure — can be overcome by well-planned projections, careful positioning of the patient and accurate X-ray beam alignment. Some relevant aspects of radiographic technique are covered by the following examples.

POSITIONING

Lung fields

The postero-anterior projection of the chest requires forward positioning of the scapulae, clear of the lung fields. (Obliquity of the peripheral X-rays makes a PA projection more effective on this point, than an anteroposterior.)

For a lateral projection of the chest, both arms are raised above the shoulders, to avoid superimposition on the lung fields.

Cervical spine

A lateral projection of the cervical spine involves tilting the patient's head backwards to clear the mandible from the upper vertebral bodies, and depressing the shoulders to prevent their superimposition on the lower vertebrae.

For an anteroposterior projection of the upper cervical vertebrae (1–3) superimposition by the mandible is prevented by the patient's mouth being open. The lower border of the upper incisor teeth (or the alveolar process of the maxilla, if the patient is edentulous) should be aligned with the lower border of the occipital bone (Fig. 24a).

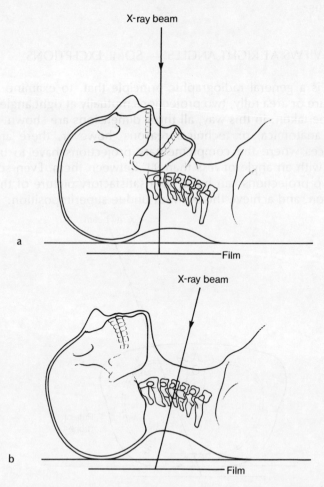

Fig. 24 Anteroposterior projections of the cervical vertebrae: principle of adjusting skull and mandible positions to show upper and lower regions.

An AP projection of the lower vertebrae (3–7) requires a backward tilt of the head so that the lower border of the mandible anteriorly is aligned with the lower margin of the occipital bone. (Fig. 24b)

Elbow

For a lateral projection, the elbow joint is flexed to a right angle, to move the olecranon process of the ulna clear of the humerus.

'TWO VIEWS AT RIGHT ANGLES' — SOME EXCEPTIONS

There is a general radiographic principle that, to examine a structure or area fully, two projections mutually at right angles must be taken. In this way, all three dimensions are shown.

For anatomical or technical reasons, however, there are instances where the complementary projections have to be taken with an angle of *less* than 90° between them. Even so, the two projections can build up a satisfactory picture of the situation, and achieve this without undue superimposition.

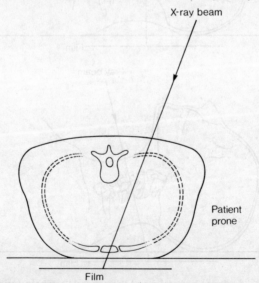

Fig. 25 Postero-anterior oblique projection of the sternum. Obliquity of the X-ray beam prevents superimposition of vertebral shadows.

Hand

The postero-anterior (dorsipalmar) projection of the hand is normally complemented by a PA Oblique (at about 45°) rather than a lateral. Otherwise, on a lateral radiograph, superimposition would obscure the 2nd–5th metacarpals.

Sternum

A true postero-anterior or anteroposterior projection of the sternum (to complement a lateral) cannot be achieved, due to superimposition by the thoracic vertebrae and mediastinal shadows. This problem is overcome by use of the PA Oblique projection, with the X-ray beam angled across the thorax (Fig. 25).

Paired structures

Lateral projections of the skull, thorax and abdomen create superimposition (right upon left) of paired structures.

Kidneys and ureters. During urography, oblique projections are normally more helpful than a lateral to clarify appearances seen on anteroposterior projections.

Ribs. A postero-anterior projection of the chest is followed up by an anteroposterior oblique projection, rather than a lateral.

Lung apices. Also clearly shown on a PA chest radiograph, these are further shown, if required, with a form of angled 'apical projection' rather than a lateral.

Mandible. Lateral oblique projections, separating right and left, are the normal complement to a postero-anterior.

THE SKULL

The cranium can be regarded as a hollow sphere. Consequently, when an X-ray beam is directed through it, some superimposition *must* occur. But the extent to which it interferes with demonstration of the various parts can be controlled by taking into account (a) the general radiopacity of structures forming the base of the skull; and (b) the relative radiolucency of the vault and, to a lesser extent, the facial skeleton.

Radiography of the skull forms a complicated but very interesting and challenging subject. The following points are only examples.

Skull vault

The anterior, posterior and side walls of the vault are readily demonstrated. The required area is placed nearer the film, and the X-ray beam is centred through the relatively radiolucent area remote from the film. Parts which adjoin the base may best be shown with the aid of a downward beam angulation — i.e., towards the base to project its denser shadow clear of the walls. (The 20° occipitofrontal projection is an example.)

Facial skeleton

Clear demonstration of the facial skeleton requires the highly radiopaque petrous temporal shadows to be projected clear of the areas of interest. Otherwise, superimposition can be a considerable problem.

The primary projection of the facial skeleton, including the paranasal air sinuses, is the *occipitomental*. The technique for this (Fig. 26) involves projecting the petrous temporal shadows below the floors of the maxillary sinuses. The facial bones are themselves superimposed only on the vault.

The facial skeleton provides a further example of how, through identically superimposing left on right, a true lateral projection has limited application. A useful projection to complement the occipitomental is the *30° occipitomental*. This extra angulation unfortunately adds to the distortion of the facial bones but offers a sufficiently different angle, for clarification of appearances seen on the basic occipitomental.

Petrous parts of the temporal bones

Despite their own radiopacity, demonstration of the petrous temporal bones also involves superimposition on radiolucent areas of the skull: on the vault, in submentovertical and 30° fronto-occipital projections; and on the areas framed by the orbital margins, in so-called 'perorbital' postero-anterior or (for greater orbit magnification) anteroposterior projections.

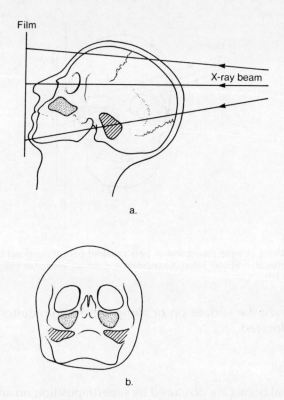

Fig. 26 Occipitomental projection of the facial skeleton: (a) relative positioning of the maxillary sinuses and petrous part of temporal bones; (b) radiographic appearance.

The petromastoid part of the temporal bone and the temporomandibular joint form yet another area for which a true lateral projection is of limited value. In this case, the solution lies in the use of a lateral oblique projection (Fig. 27). Beam angulation separates right from left and superimposes only the thin, homogeneous, squamous part of the temporal bone (remote from the film) on to the area of interest.

TANGENTIAL PROJECTIONS

Several projections are tangential in nature, if not in name. Their common principle is that the X-ray beam is directed so

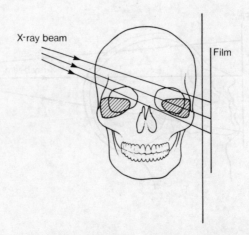

X-ray beam

Film

Fig. 27 Lateral oblique projection of petromastoid part of temporal bone and temporomandibular joint: X-ray beam angulation separates shadows of right and left.

as to graze the surface on or along which the required structure is located.

The skull

The nasal bones are obscured by superimposition on an occipitomental radiograph of the facial bones. A lateral projection shows the nasal bones clearly but, if a projection at 90° to this is required, the supero-inferior is used (Fig. 28a).

Tangential projections also show:

— an area of the vault where a depressed fracture is suspected
— the zygomatic arches (submentovertical and 30° fronto-occipital projections)
— the mastoid processes of the temporal bones.

Thoracic cage

The X-ray beam is tangential to the wall of the thoracic cage for:

— a lateral projection of a scapula
— an inferosuperior projection of a clavicle.

Upper limb

Surface features of the humerus shown in this way are:

— the bicipital groove
— the ulnar groove
— tuberosities (to show tendon insertions).

A tangential projection shows the carpal tunnel of a hyper-extended wrist (Fig. 28d).

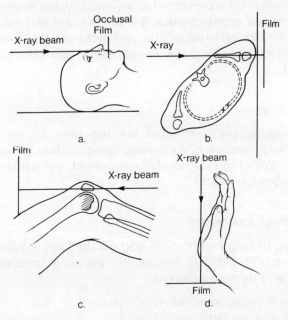

Fig. 28 Tangential projections (a) supero-inferior of nasal bones; (b) lateral of scapula; (c) inferosuperior of patella; (d) inferosuperior of carpal tunnel.

Lower limb

Tangential projections of the knee region show:

— the superior tibiofibular joint (oblique projection)
— the patella (inferosuperior) (Fig. 28c)
— the intercondylar notch of the femur.

The calcaneus is obscured by superimposition on dorsi-plantar projections of the foot and an anteroposterior of the ankle. An angled axial projection, clearing its shadow from the adjacent tarsal bones, complements a lateral projection.

A tangential projection shows the sesamoid bones at the plantar aspect of the metatarsal heads.

AUTOTOMOGRAPHY

This term has come into use to describe techniques in which superimposition is prevented or lessened by *movement during a lengthened exposure time*. It is *not* the case that the patient is simply 'allowed to move': the part of the patient which forms 'the object' must be *firmly immobilised*; only *other* parts are moved.

Cervical spine

The 'moving jaw' technique may be used for an antero-posterior projection of the cervical spine, to show all seven vertebrae. With the skull firmly immobilised, the patient opens and closes the mouth.

'Breathing' techniques

Blurring of lung and possibly also rib shadows is achieved by allowing (rather than instructing) the patient to breathe gently, for clearer demonstration of:

— the thoracic spine (lateral projection)
— the scapula (anteroposterior)
— lumbar vertebrae (anteroposterior)
— the sternum (postero-anterior oblique)
— an injured humerus, immobilised by the patient's side ('transthoracic' lateral projection).

Suggested exercise

— A series of radiographs, including projections mentioned above, should be studied to see the effects of manoeuvres to minimise superimposition.

Related studies

When encountering and learning radiographic techniques, as their training proceeds, students should learn to recognise features designed to minimise superimposition.

Students will be aided in learning the spatial relationships between bony structures, by close study of an articulated skeleton.

16

How do standard projections enable image distortion to be minimised?

Distortion is said to have occurred when the *shape of the image* does not correspond to the *shape of the object*. There are two separate causes:

foreshortening happens when the object plane is *not* approached by the X-ray beam *at right angles*;
elongation occurs when the object plane does *not lie parallel* to the film.

ADJUSTMENT OF THE PATIENT'S POSITION

It is normal practice, with conventional equipment, for the X-ray beam to be directed towards the film, at right angles. This arrangement enables the focus-film distance to be measured accurately, and raises no problem if a secondary radiation grid is in use.

If it is possible, *the patient's position is adjusted* to bring the object plane to lie at right angles to the X-ray beam. Thus, foreshortening does not occur (although it must be remembered, especially when a large field is used, that the rays become more oblique away from the centre), and — because the object plane is then parallel to the film — elongation is also avoided.

Examples of adjusting the patient's position to fit this standard 90° relationship between X-ray beam and film, include:

Hip joint

The technique for an anteroposterior projection of the hip joint requires slight internal rotation or, at least, a 'neutral' (anatomical) position of the leg, to bring the femoral neck at right angles to the X-ray beam (see Fig. 29).

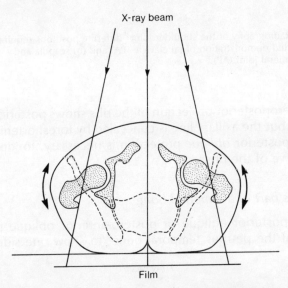

Fig. 29 Anteroposterior projections of the hip joints (diagrammatic cross-section through pelvis): internal and external limb rotation influences foreshortening of femoral neck shadows.

Shoulder region

From the position in which the patient directly faces the X-ray tube, there has to be an appreciable degree of rotation to bring the plane of the scapula at 90° to the X-ray beam for an anteroposterior projection of the scapula or to show the glenohumeral joint (Fig. 30b).

Rotation in the *opposite* direction is required to bring the mean axis of the *clavicle* at 90° to the beam for either a postero-anterior or (if the patient's condition dictates) an anteroposterior projection. See Figure 30a.

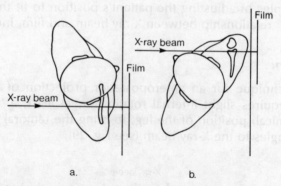

a.   b.

Fig. 30 Radiography of the shoulder joint: differing positions required for undistorted demonstration of (a) clavicle (PA) and (b) scapula and glenohumeral joint (AP).

Ribs

An anteroposterior projection of the ribs shows posterior parts clearly but the axillary line is concealed by foreshortening. An anteroposterior *oblique* projection is necessary, to 'open up' the curve of the ribs.

Petrous part of a temporal bone

Anteroposterior oblique or postero-anterior oblique projections of the petrous temporal bone (to show one side only)

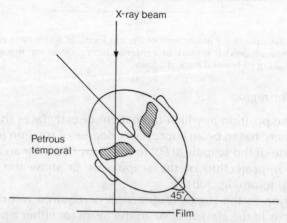

Fig. 31 Oblique projections of petrous part of temporal bone: principle of rotation to bring object parallel to film.

require rotation of the skull to bring the petrous ridge at 90° to the X-ray beam (Fig. 31).

Joint spaces, foramina and fractures

Radiographic demonstration of a *foramen* lying within a bone, requires one simple condition to be fulfilled: that the X-ray beam is projected *along the foramen's axis*. Otherwise, the image of the lumen is foreshortened (from a circle to an ellipse, for example).

The same principle applies to the demonstration of a *joint space* or a *bone fracture*: any obliquity will tend to narrow or even conceal the space between the adjoining bony margins.

Oblique projections frequently remedy the shortcomings of standard anteroposterior and lateral projections. Examples include:

— the *optic foramina*
— *intervertebral foramina*, usually in the cervical or lumbar regions of the spine (see Fig. 32b)
— *sacro-iliac joints* (Fig. 33)
— *sternoclavicular joints* (Fig. 34)
— a *pars interarticularis* of a lumbar vertebra's neural arch (Fig. 32a) which can be the site of a bony defect (spondylolysis).

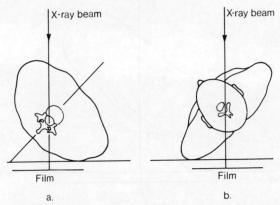

Fig. 32 Oblique projections of the vertebrae: (a) lumbar, to show pars interarticularis; and (b) cervical to show intervertebral foramen.

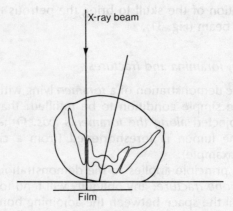

Fig. 33 Oblique projection of sacro-iliac joints (cross-section through pelvis): rotation to align joint plane with X-ray beam.

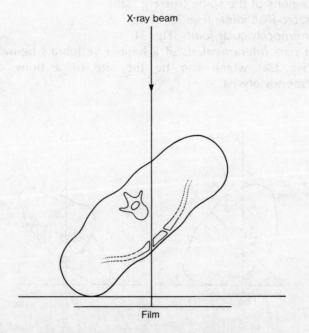

Fig. 34 Postero-anterior oblique projection of sternoclavicular joints: rotation to align joint space with X-ray beam.

Vertebral column

For lateral projections, positioning of the patient with the median plane parallel to the film is necessary for showing the intervertebral disc spaces clearly.

For an anteroposterior projection of the lumbar spine, the positioning procedure is designed to reduce the natural curvature (which, in contrast to the thoracic curvature, tends to be adverse to the divergent X-ray beam) so that the intervertebral disc spaces can be shown clearly. The supine patient's shoulders are raised slightly and the hips and knees are flexed (Fig. 35).

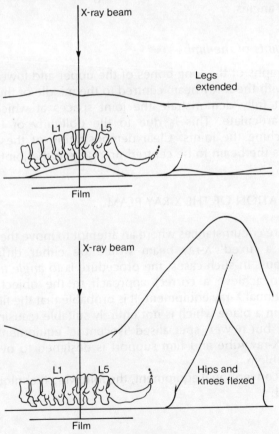

Fig. 35 Anteroposterior projection of lumbar vertebrae: reduction of curvature by adjustment of patient's position.

Hands

The routine postero-anterior projection of the hands becomes unsatisfactory when there is an arthritic condition causing flexion of the fingers. In such cases, an anteroposterior projection improves alignment between the joint spaces and the divergent X-ray beam.

Feet

Demonstration of the intertarsal and tarsometatarsal joints is clearer on a dorsiplantar oblique projection (rather than a simple DP) — the X-ray beam meeting the dorsum of the foot at right angles.

Main joints of the limbs

Radiographs of the long bones of the upper and lower limbs, taken with the X-ray beam centred to the middle of the shafts, will not fully demonstrate the joint spaces at which these bones articulate. This is due to the obliquity of the rays approaching the joints. Clear demonstration of these joints requires the beam to be centred precisely to the joint plane.

ANGULATION OF THE X-RAY BEAM

There are circumstances where an attempt to move the patient to suit a 'fixed' X-ray beam would be either difficult or dangerous. In such cases, the procedure is to *angle the X-ray beam* to achieve a correct approach to the object. Using conventional X-ray equipment, it is probable that the film must remain in a plane which is not entirely suitable (causing elongation); but newer, specialised 'isocentric' equipment with a linked X-ray tube and film support is designed to overcome this problem.

With conventional equipment, the following techniques may be used:

Sacrum

Anteroposterior projections of the *sacrum* and *lumbosacral articulation* are achieved without foreshortening when the X-ray beam is angled cephalad. Although this creates some elongation, a compensatory adjustment of the patient's position, instead, would be difficult to achieve.

Cervical spine

For an anteroposterior projection of the *lower cervical vertebrae* (3rd–7th), slight cephalad angulation of the X-ray beam demonstrates clear intervertebral spaces. The patient's

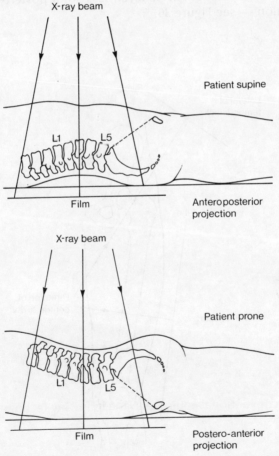

Fig. 36 Comparative alignment of X-ray beam to pelvis for anteroposterior and postero-anterior projections of the abdomen. Dotted line shows pelvic inlet.

position, in this case, is designed to reduce superimposition — but the backward tilt of the head tends to increase the slope of the cervical spine (see Fig. 24b).

Pelvic canal

Angulation of the X-ray beam along the axis of the pelvic canal enables the urinary bladder and other pelvic structures to be shown clearly. It should be noted that the X-ray beam does not pass along this axis when either an anteroposterior projection is taken of the abdomen or (even less so) a postero-anterior projection — see Figure 36.

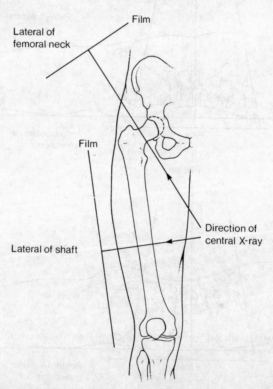

Fig. 37 Lateral projections of the femur: different angulations required to prevent foreshortening.

Femoral neck

For a *horizontal beam lateral* projection of the *femoral neck*, the X-ray beam is projected at 90° to the axis of the neck to prevent foreshortening. This angle should be noted in comparison with the technique for a lateral projection of the femoral shaft (see Fig. 37).

This is a case where the film can be positioned parallel to the object, to prevent elongation.

Fluid

The *presence of fluid* (if clinically significant) can be demonstrated in the body when the X-ray beam is directed along the fluid/gas interface (or, it may be preferred to say, at 90° to the plane intersecting this interface). There is thus a requirement for the X-ray beam to be *horizontal*.

This simple fact must be remembered especially when the patient's illness prevents standard positions and projections from being obtained. The 'object' is the fluid/gas interface; foreshortening may conceal its presence but elongation cannot — although surrounding anatomical shadows may be distorted.

Suggested exercise

— A series of radiographs, including projections mentioned above, should be studied to see the effects of moves to minimise distortion.

Related studies

When encountering and learning radiographic techniques, as their training proceeds, students should recognise features designed to minimise distortion.

Students will be aided in learning the spatial relationships between bony structures, by close study of an articulated skeleton.

17

Why are diagnostic X-ray tubes equipped with rotating anodes?

Some X-ray tubes have *stationary (fixed)* anodes. The target is a rectangular block of tungsten embedded in the sloping face of a cylindrical copper anode. Although they produce X-rays quite satisfactorily for a few purposes, these tubes are only rarely found in use in diagnostic X-ray departments.

Compared with a stationary anode tube, a *rotating* anode X-ray tube (Fig. 38) is more expensive, more bulky, and has moving parts which wear with use. There must, therefore, be a good reason why, despite these points, it is generally preferred.

The explanation stems from the fact that radiographic exposures need to be *short*. An exposure is the product of an exposure *time* and a *rate* of X-ray production. Thus, any method of increasing the rate consequently reduces the required time — and the risk of movement during the exposure.

The rate is usually expressed in terms of the average tube current (mA) — i.e., the average rate at which electric charge flows through the tube. (It is also affected by the value of the kilovoltage across the tube but it is assumed that other image criteria determine the selected kV.) There is no limit, through their own properties, to the rate at which X-rays may be produced. But bombardment of the tube target by electrons

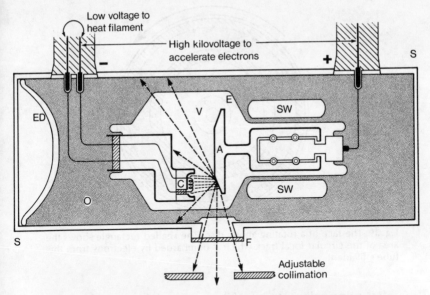

Fig. 38 A rotating anode X-ray tube. Key: (A) anode; (C) cathode; (E) envelope; (V) vacuum; (SW) stator windings; (O) oil; (ED) expansion diaphragm; (F) aluminium filter; (S) shield.

is responsible for producing *heat* as well as X-rays — and there *is* a limit to the permissible rate of heat production. This is imposed by the need to prevent or, at least, restrict thermal damage to the X-ray tube target.

When electrons bombard the target, its temperature begins to rise. The rate at which this rise takes place depends on three factors:

— the heat capacity of the target
— the rate of cooling
— the rate of heating (product of tube current and kilovoltage).

Heat capacity

The larger the target's heat capacity, the lower is the temperature rise resulting from each unit of heat produced. Expressed in an alternative way: the larger the heat capacity, the higher is the rate at which heat may be produced, for a given temperature rise.

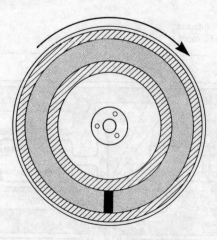

Fig. 39 The face of a rotating anode disc. The shaded rectangle shows the area of the circular focal track which is bombarded by electrons from the tube's filament.

It is principally in terms of its very much larger heat capacity, that a rotating anode shows its advantage. The area of a stationary anode within which the heat is produced, coincides exactly with the area of X-ray production — i.e., the target. In a rotating anode X-ray tube, however, the rapidly rotating disc continuously presents a changing area, the **focal track**, for heating by the electron beam. Despite this, the area of X-ray production remains constant, and equally small as a stationary anode (see Fig. 39).

This increased *loading area* of a rotating anode, compared with a stationary anode, very greatly increases the permitted rate at which heat — *and X-rays* — may be produced.

Cooling rate

The rate at which cooling occurs is also greater for a rotating anode. Direct comparison between rotating and stationary anode cooling rates is difficult because different methods are employed. The stationary target cools principally by conduction to the mass of the copper anode; the focal track of a rotating disc loses heat firstly by conduction to the whole anode disc, and then almost entirely by radiation. The design of the anode — with the disc mounted on a narrow stem —

discourages loss by conduction, since the spread of heat to the moving parts of the rotation mechanism could slow down and eventually prevent rotation. This would cause damage to the focal track since, at a slower rotational speed, the reduced spread of heat would lead to a greater temperature rise.

The speed of rotation is important. In an 'ordinary' tube, it is of the order of 3000 revolutions per minute. So-called 'high-speed' anodes have speeds of around 9000 r.p.m., or even higher, to increase still further the safe rate at which X-rays may be produced. Higher rotational speeds are not achieved without difficulty: some form of braking needs to be incorporated to come into use after an exposure, to reduce mechanical stresses; and the rotation apparatus itself acts as a source of heat.

An illustration of these points may be observed in some X-ray equipment when, during fluoroscopy, the anode is not rotated. If the modest heating rate of a fluoroscopic tube current does not threaten the thermal safety of the anode, the disc may remain stationary until, in preparation for exposure of a radiograph, it is made to rotate, to cope with the heat accompanying the required high rate of X-ray production.

Suggested exercises

— Students will be familiar with the noise of an anode rotating. Comparison might be made between the various tubes in use in the X-ray department to see if there is any correlation between the age of the tube and its noise and the length of the 'run-out' time.
— If a tube offers different anode rotation speeds for the radiographers' use, it may be interesting to compare the maximum permissible values and combinations of kilovoltage, current (mA) and exposure time which each speed will allow for a given focal spot size.

Related studies

X-ray tube design and construction; tube rating.

18

Why does a diagnostic X-ray tube usually have *two* focal spots?

One of the radiographer's concerns is to minimise image unsharpness. A dual-focus X-ray tube is the standard piece of equipment used in diagnostic radiography. Usually, the two foci are different in size: the larger being referred to as the **broad** focus; the smaller, as the **fine** focus. Each has its own particular purpose.

Use of the 'broad' focus

The broad focus has a higher heat capacity than the fine focus — i.e., the width, and possibly the length, of its focal track on the anode disc is larger. Thus, for a given temperature rise (from room temperature up to a calculated safe maximum) heat — and, therefore, X-rays — can be produced at a higher rate than when the fine focus is in use.

Movement of the patient during the exposure can be a cause of image unsharpness. An obvious method of keeping this to a minimum is to shorten exposure time. But this step cannot be undertaken unless the *quantity* of X-rays required to produce a satisfactory image remains the same. Quantity is the product of *rate* and *time*. Consequently, if time is to be reduced, the rate must be proportionately increased.

Thus, under circumstances when *movement during the*

exposure is anticipated (despite attempts to prevent it) the use of broad focus and the shorter exposure times which it allows, will minimise the risk of movement unsharpness.

Use of the 'fine' focus

The fact that the X-rays do *not* emanate from a *point source* causes all X-ray shadows to be surrounded by an incomplete shadow, or *penumbra*. This is recorded on an image as geometric unsharpness (Fig. 40).

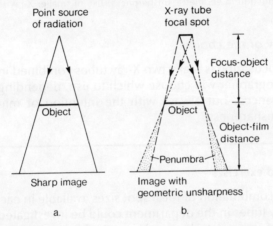

Fig. 40 Radiographic image formation with (a) an ideal (theoretical) radiation source, and (b) a practical source.

The fine focus of an X-ray tube creates a smaller penumbra than does the broad focus (Fig. 41). It also, however, has a smaller heat capacity (the fine focal track on the anode disc being narrower than the broad).

The maximum permitted rate of heat and X-ray production — both governed by the tube current (mA) — is, therefore, lower. Consequently, for a given quantity of X-rays needed for exposing a radiograph, the required exposure time must be greater.

Thus, use of the fine focus (compared with the broad focus) will reduce penumbra and — provided that the object can be immobilised during the exposure — may reduce image unsharpness.

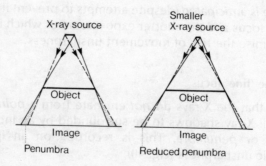

Fig. 41 Reduction in geometric unsharpness: use of smaller X-ray source.

Summary of the choice

A dual-focus tube is really two X-ray tubes combined into one. The radiographer will choose which to use, depending on the circumstances, but always with the intention of minimising image unsharpness.

Suggested exercises

— The combination of focal spot sizes available in each of the X-ray tubes in the department could be investigated. It may be of interest to learn why particular combinations were chosen when a tube was bought — and for which radiographic examinations they are routinely used.

— Bearing in mind that the terms 'broad' and 'fine' are only relative and not absolute, it will be interesting for students to construct a simple table of figures for any X-ray tube to show the maximum permitted tube kilovoltage and current (mA) combinations at a series of exposure times (0.01 s, 0.05 s, 0.1 s, 0.2 s, 0.5 s, etc.) for each focus.

Related studies

X-ray tube design and construction; tube rating.

19

Why are secondary radiation grids used?

Purpose of a grid

The X-ray beam emerging from the patient comprises:

1. transmitted primary radiation conveying information about the object
2. secondary radiation, or 'scatter', emitted from irradiated structures. This does not represent information about the object; its effect on the image is to reduce contrast.

A grid is used to remove from the X-ray beam approaching the film, a significant proportion of the scatter, while allowing a high proportion of the primary beam to pass, unhindered. A grid thus tends to enhance image contrast.

Mode of action

A grid is able to serve its purpose through differences in the direction of primary and secondary radiation.

Primary radiation travels in straight lines, diverging from the X-ray tube target.

Secondary radiation also travels in straight lines but its direction is random.

A grid is a thin, plate-like structure. It is composed of a parallel series of thin strips of material, alternately *radiolucent*

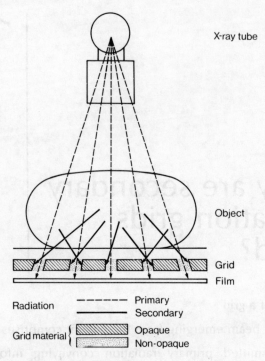

X-ray tube

Object

Grid
Film

Radiation ------- Primary
Secondary

Grid material { Opaque
Non-opaque

Fig. 42 Reduction in the amount of scatter (secondary radiation) reaching the film. Cross section through grid (diagrammatic) to show its selective action.

(aluminium or plastic) and *radiopaque* (lead). It provides (Fig. 42) a set of channels or spaces which allow free passage of aligned radiation, but whose walls absorb radiation not so aligned.

The cross-sectional dimensions of the radiolucent spaces are important. The relationship between *height* and *width* of a space is termed the **grid ratio**. This determines (Fig. 43) how effectively oblique scattered radiation is prevented from passing through the grid. A high-ratio grid will only allow through narrow-angle scatter which approximates to the direction of primary radiation.

Types of grid

The simplest form of grid has its opaque strips precisely **parallel**

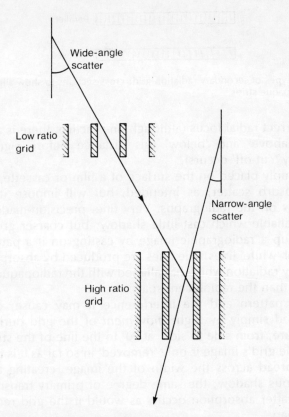

Fig. 43 Grid ratio relates the 'height' of a radiolucent interspace to its width. An increase in grid ratio reduces the permitted angular difference between primary X-rays and scatter, before absorption occurs.

to each other. This arrangement imposes few conditions on its use but creates a problem of misalignment between oblique primary rays and the radiolucent spaces through which they must pass.

This problem is overcome by a progressive inward tilting of the opaque strips, at increasing distances from the grid's centre line, so that the spaces maintain full alignment to all primary rays. This arrangement (Fig. 44) forms a **focused** grid, which is more favourable than a parallel grid to the transmission of primary X-rays but requires to be used in a more precise manner: (i) with the X-ray beam centred to its midline; (ii) its strips converging towards the X-ray tube; (iii) the tube target at

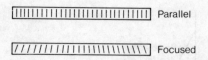

Fig. 44 Types of secondary radiation grid: cross-sections to show alignment of the opaque strips.

the correct radial focus (although, in practice, there is a tolerance 'above' and 'below' this distance before significant primary 'cut-off' occurs).

If simply placed on the surface of a film or cassette, a grid will absorb scatter, as intended, but will impose its own shadow on the radiographs. Very fine, precision-made grids are available which cast little shadow; but coarser grids will break up a radiographic image by casting on it a pattern of parallel 'white' lines. The lines are produced by absorption of primary radiation which has aligned with the radiopaque strips rather than the radiolucent spaces.

This pattern and the interference it may cause, can be removed simply by slight *movement* of the grid during the exposure, from side to side, at 90° to the line of the strips. In fact, the grid's image is only 'removed' in so far as it is blurred and spread across the width of the image, creating a homogeneous shadow; the same degree of primary transmission and scatter absorption occurs as would if the grid remained stationary.

Grid movement is achieved by its being mounted in a frame positioned between the film plane and table top or other work surface. This arrangement is generally known as a **bucky**, in honour of one of its inventors.

The conventional grid, with a single set of parallel lines, offers no opposition to the scatter directed *along* rather than *across* its spaces. Assuming an equal spatial distribution, approximately 50% of the scatter will therefore pass through a grid, unhindered. If this amount proves sufficient to keep image contrast unacceptably low, a *crossed*, or *cross-hatch* grid can be used. This consists of two grids, one on top of the other, with their lines arranged mutually at 90° — one set transverse, one longitudinal.

Such an arrangement can be set up, if a situation demands,

by the radiographer with, for example, a grid cassette used in conjunction with a bucky grid.

Disadvantages of using a grid

1. Through its inevitable absorption of primary radiation, a grid requires an *increased* quantity of radiation to be used in creating a radiographic image.

The term, **grid factor**, expresses the order of this increase — being the ratio between the larger quantity of radiation required to produce an image when a grid is used, and the smaller quantity when it is not.

This need for an exposure increase brings two significant disadvantages:

    a. the radiation hazard to the patient is increased
    b. the likelihood of movement during the exposure time is increased.

2. When a grid is used, the radiographer is able to angle the X-ray beam only *along* the line of the grid spaces, not across. If a crossed grid is used, the central X-ray must be perpendicular to the grid.

3. A grid movement mechanism requires a greater separation between object and film, so tending to increase geometric unsharpness.

Criteria for use of a grid

The decision whether, in the light of its disadvantages, to use a grid, must be made according to the diagnostic value of the image.

If it is considered that the image without a grid will have such poor contrast that its value in diagnosing the patient's condition will only be slight, it will be in the patient's interests to use a grid.

If, however, the diagnostic purpose of a radiograph is expected to be met, despite the effects of scattered radiation, or where the risk of increased movement unsharpness poses more of a problem than loss of contrast, it will be to the patient's benefit to *omit* a grid.

There are many radiographic examinations for which the decision, to use a grid or not, is clear-cut. But there are others (chest, shoulder, cervical spine) where the radiographer must make a decision after evaluating the circumstances, rather than simply following the routine.

Suggested exercises

— Students should investigate the types of grid that are in use in the X-ray department: what are the grid ratios and methods of movement?

— An old, partly dismantled or dissected grid should be inspected to see precisely the dimensions and pattern of its construction.

— Test radiographs of phantoms should be exposed with and without the use of a grid, and then compared.

Related studies

Grid construction; types of grid; movements; uses.

20

Why are special storage arrangements provided for X-ray films?

All photographic emulsions have a limited *'shelf life'*. Students may have seen printed on unexposed film boxes that the manufacturers stipulate *expiry dates* before which the film must be used; and advise storage in a cool place before exposure.

The fixing of an expiry date is due to the tendency for changes to occur spontaneously within an emulsion. These make unexposed silver halide crystals developable — and their visible effect on a processed radiographic is of a density in areas which have received no exposure. Thus, *image contrast is reduced*.

The rate at which these changes occur, tends to increase with temperature; and their effect accumulates with age. It is thus ideal for films to be *stored in a cool place* and *used without undue delay*, after delivery from the manufacturer.

Manufacturers specify expiry dates, to mark the end of periods during which, if correctly stored, film will show no sign of deterioration.

Length of storage

It is reasonable to assume that the film manufacturer can deliver any required quantity of film promptly to the X-ray department as required (if not, another manufacturer will take over!). The rate at which films need to be ordered will, therefore, be determined by the rate at which they are used. Careful record-keeping in the X-ray department shows how many boxes of each size of film are used per week. The regular order placed with the manufacturer will thus be a replacement delivery to match.

The unusual chance of a delayed film delivery needs to be considered, however. A reserve stock of film is maintained as a precaution.

It is usual for the rate of film usage in a department to continue to be monitored, rather than regarded as 'static'. Patterns of usage of each film size can change, as radiographic techniques are modified.

The film store

Provision of a 'cool' room even in a centrally-heated X-ray department should not be difficult. The temperature should be consistently below 20 °C, if possible; there must be no direct sunshine heating the room, and there must be some form of ventilation.

Ideal storage involves other external factors, however, apart from temperature:

— The room should be away from radiographic examination rooms and, if considered necessary, have some form of radiation protection incorporated in its walls.
— The site of the storeroom must not be inconveniently remote from darkrooms and film dispensers (cassette loading machines).
— Shelving must be provided, for film boxes to be stored 'on-end' (rather than stacked flat). This arrangement tends to prevent physical damage (which, if severe, can create developable marks in an emulsion) and aids a 'rotational' system of usage: the oldest boxes being used first.
— Although films are sealed in moistureproof wrapping, it is advisable for the storeroom to be completely dry and well ventilated to prevent any dampness or chemical fumes penetrating the film boxes. (Processing chemicals should not be stored with films, in case leakages occur).

Storage in the darkroom

After being fetched from the storeroom, a box of films will be opened and loaded into a special drawer, known as a 'hopper'. This has a curved floor which, despite their varying sizes, keeps the top edges of all films up to the same convenient level.

Once films reach the darkroom hopper (or a dispensing machine), the storage safety priorities change. Time is no longer relevant — the films are soon to be used; the temperature will be that prevailing in the room; and there will already be protection against X-radiation. Now out of their wrapping, films need to be protected against (1) physical damage — rough handling, scratches, wet or greasy finger-marks — and (2) exposure to 'white' light.

Careful handling technique — touching film *edges* only — minimises the risk of artefacts.

In a machine, protection against light is ensured. In a darkroom hopper, a pressure-operated switch breaks the white light circuit when the hopper is opened.

Cassette storage

Finally, mention should be made of how films are stored in cassettes, awaiting exposure. The main risk is from unintentional exposure to X-rays. Cassettes should be stored in protected hatches or boxes, rather than left lying in places where they may be accidentally exposed.

Suggested exercises

— Students should find out how the rate of film usage is monitored in the X-ray department.
— It will be of interest, also to learn (i) how regularly film orders are placed; and (ii) how much reserve stock is left, in the event of a delivery being delayed.
— Students should see how the departmental storeroom provides the required conditions, and how a rotational usage system is implemented.
— It might prove interesting to store a single film in a light-

proof envelope, away from X-radiation but otherwise in adverse storage conditions, for a period of weeks or months, before processing it, to see the deterioration that has occurred.

Related studies

Film storage conditions; record keeping.

21

Why are silver recovery systems operated?

Photographic film emulsions contain **silver** in the form of **halide** crystals — i.e., as salts formed by combination with some elements of the 'halogen' group.

Exposure and development cause a number of the silver halide crystals — those which form the image pattern — to change into metallic silver. The remainder serve no purpose and are removed by fixation. During its use, therefore, a fixer solution accumulates a concentration of silver which is of no further photographic use.

Silver is a scarce world resource of high value. It is not, therefore, a commodity to be (literally) poured down the drain when a spent fixer solution is discarded. Instead, it is reclaimed as fully as possible and sold by the hospital, to offset some of the initial film costs. The reclaimed silver then enters a recycling path — some of it, no doubt, being bought by film manufacturers.

Thus the principal reasons for silver recovery concern economics and conservation.

Recovery from fixer solution

Either of two methods may be used:

Electrolytic

An electrolytic method makes use of the electrical conductivity of a fixer solution. The application of a potential difference across a certain volume of the solution causes a current to flow in the form of negative ions travelling to the anode(s), and positive ions, including the silver, to the cathode. Metallic silver is deposited, or 'plated out', at the cathode. Efficient operation of an electrolytic silver recovery unit, involves a careful matching of the electric current to the concentration of silver ions between the electrodes. Slow, natural convection currents at room temperature safely allow a low rate of recovery. Increased rates usually require forced circulation within the tank to prevent electrolysis of fixer chemicals and consequent contamination of the solution.

Electrolysis provides a clean, non-destructive method of silver recovery: the fixer solution may be re-used for photographic purposes.

Metal exchange (replacement)

Metal exchange (replacement) methods employ the electrochemical properties of metals, whereby a metal in solution can be plated by reaction with a solid form of another metal (higher up the 'electrochemical series').

This then, itself, goes into solution, exchanging places with the recovered metal.

The method is usually implemented by slow passage of silver-laden fixer solution through iron 'wool'. The method is 'destructive', since the treated, iron-laden effluent has no photographic use.

Metal exchange methods can be also be carried out by commercial metal dealers on discarded fixer solution, collected from X-ray departments. In some cases the fixer undergoes both electrolytic and metal exchange treatments to ensure full recovery of the available silver.

Recovery from discarded radiographs

Radiographs usually have only a limited life — in the sense that their medical value during the management of a patient's illness is reduced or disappears as the patient recovers. Even so, all radiographs are stored for a statutory number of years to satisfy medico-legal requirements.

At the end of this period, radiographs are discarded. Recovery of the silver, of which the radiographic images have been composed, is then possible. This is entirely a commercial process on radiographs collected from the X-ray departments.

Suggested exercises

— Students should investigate the methods of silver recovery used in their X-ray departments, enquiring

why these are preferred to any other systems that are available
how they are managed and checked (daily or weekly)
what financial return the X-ray department receives.

Related studies

Silver recovery methods and equipment.

22

What are 'exposure factors'?

Details of how to position the X-ray tube, patient and film, are not, alone, sufficient to specify the technique for a radiographic projection; further technical data are required, commonly termed the *exposure factors*:

— kilovoltage (peak value) applied across the X-ray tube
— X-ray tube current (milliamperes)
— exposure time (seconds)
— focus-film distance
— size of tube focus
— type of film
— type of intensifying screens
— secondary radiation grid data.

These factors are variously chosen for a radiographic projection, according to:

Radiopacity of the object to be penetrated by the X-ray beam

This takes into account an object's thickness (i.e., the dimension traversed by the X-ray beam), its density and effective atomic number.

The extent to which the X-ray beam is required to penetrate

110

an object is determined by the part which causes maximum attenuation — often loosely referred to as its 'densest' part.

The exposure factor which provides this required penetration, or beam energy, is the *tube kilovoltage*.

Required (photographic) density and contrast of the image

Confirmation that radiation has penetrated an object is provided by the densities which appear on a radiograph. These must be sufficiently high to form a full image, with every component part identifiable. Thus a sufficient *quantity* of radiation must reach the X-ray film.

The quantity of radiation *required* for radiography of a given object depends (as well as on its own attenuating effect) on the *speed* of the *film* and *intensifying screens*.

The *provision* of this required amount is achieved, potentially, by several factors. Principally, the *tube current* (mA) and *exposure time* are adjusted to vary the quantity of radiation to which a film is exposed.

Their product, *milliampere-seconds* (mAs), measures the quantity of electric charge crossing the X-ray tube during an exposure.

In some X-ray departments, it is the practice for separate values of tube current (*mA*) and exposure time(*s*) to be stipulated for a given radiographic projection. When the length of the exposure time is particularly relevant — for an 'autotomography' technique, for instance — this separation is useful.

At other times, however, the practice of quoting only a *milliampere-seconds* value may be better. It is then left to the radiographer's skill, to select a particular mA value and exposure time which make best use of a generator's power and X-ray tube's capacity. Many generators, in fact, offer only the choice of an mAs value — determination of tube current being under automatic electronic control.

Also to be considered are the *focus-film distance, tube kilovoltage* and, if used, a *secondary radiation grid*. But these three factors are usually determined for independent reasons; their effect on the radiation quantity requirement is consequential.

Every part of an object should be shown on the image, *contrasting* with its surroundings. The exposure factors mainly determining this are the tube *kilovoltage* and, if required, a *secondary radiation grid*.

In that contrast is the difference between image *densities*, it is arguable that all the exposure factors which influence density, also have a bearing on contrast.

Minimisation of unsharpness

Every exposure factor listed above has a potential effect on eventual image unsharpness.

Geometric. When unsharpness is likely to arise from geometric causes, these can be decreased by a *focal spot size* reduction, and a *focus-film distance* increase.

Photographic. If photographic influences predominate, unsharpness can be lessened by reducing the speed of both *film* and *intensifying screens*.

Movement. The risk of movement during an exposure may be lessened by *increasing* film and screen speed, focal spot size and tube kilovoltage; and *reducing* focus-film distance and grid factor (or omitting a grid).

Radiation protection

It is difficult to exclude any exposure factor from having an effect on the radiation hazard to the patient.

A direct effect results from the *speed of the image recording system*, the *focus-film distance, tube kilovoltage*, and *grid factor* (or whether one is used, at all).

Indirectly, a favourable focal spot size and short exposure time, by contributing to an image's diagnostic value, may lessen the need for further exposure.

'Setting' exposure factors

The procedure of 'setting' exposure factors can, particularly for an inexperienced student radiographer, occupy more than just a few moments. If this follows positioning and, during this time, the patient is allowed to move at all from the precise, required position, the value of the radiograph may be in doubt.

Whenever possible, exposure factors for a projection should

be set — even if only approximately, pending closer examination of the patient — *before* positioning. In this way, only a final check or adjustment will be necessary, and the delay between positioning and exposure will be minimal.

Suggested exercises

— Students should investigate the exposure factor tables which may be in use in an X-ray department or, equally, the pre-set automated programmes for projections of various parts of the body. Connections should be traced between the factors selected and the criteria outlined above.

(It will very probably be found that factors for identical projections will vary between radiographic rooms. Such variations are accounted for by differences in the type and age of X-ray generators and tubes. A consistency should still be found within the set of factors stipulated for any single equipment.)

23

Why do radiographers adjust the tube kilovoltage?

Radiographers may have four matters in mind when selecting the kV value for any given projection: penetration of the object; image contrast; image unsharpness; and radiation protection.

Penetration

The extent to which an object needs to be penetrated by the X-ray beam, is determined by the object's natural 'densest part' — i.e., the part which, by virtue of its composition, causes maximum attenuation of the radiation (excepting some metallic parts and opaque contrast agents). If this structure is not distinguishable from its surroundings, the diagnostic value of a radiograph may not be complete.

The point might be mentioned that 'the object' is not necessarily the whole structure being radiographed. Its 'densest part' has thus to be considered according to the diagnostic purpose of a radiograph.

Examples

Skull
Submentovertical and 30° fronto-occipital projections are both employed to demonstrate the base of the skull. For

114

this purpose, the range 70–85 kVp might be used. Both projections, however, can *also* be used to show, in profile, the *zygomatic arches*. In this case — when the zygomatic arch is the 'object', rather than the base of the skull — the required penetration is much less, and perhaps 55–65 kVp would be selected.

Shoulder

A similar reduction of kVp is made when an anteroposterior projection of the shoulder is intended to show the acromioclavicular joint. The 'ordinary' kVp for an AP shoulder gives penetration of the glenohumeral joint. For the acromioclavicular joint, however, 10–15 kVp less is selected.

Image contrast

If ensuring penetration of the object were the only aim governing kilovoltage selection, it would seem reasonable for a single, constant, high kV value to be used for *all* projections — sufficient for the densest part of *any* object to be penetrated. But this is not so. There are two reasons why not:

1. Assuming that the object has been satisfactorily penetrated, the difference between attenuation coefficients for the various body tissues *decreases* as radiation energy *increases*. Thus, the range of radiation intensities transmitted through the object becomes less as the kVp is raised. Consequently, image contrast is reduced.

2. Additionally, as the kVp is increased, the direction of the *scattered radiation* becomes more 'forward' and its average energy becomes greater; thus more scatter tends to reach the film, reducing image contrast. A secondary radiation grid will lessen this effect but cannot eliminate it.

Optimum kilovoltage

This term, sometimes used, is defined as the kV at which the X-radiation *just* penetrates the most radiopaque, natural part of the object. The optimum kV thus creates (i) the widest range of transmitted radiation intensities, and (ii) the lowest proportion of scattered radiation incident on the film. It therefore produces the greatest image contrast.

This concept of an 'optimum kV' tends to be theoretical rather than practical, however. Precise determination of its value would require a degree of experimentation which, with a hospital patient, is obviously unacceptable. In practice, therefore, a radiographer estimates a kVp value within a range which, from experience, is known to achieve penetration of the object but not go so far as to produce very poor image contrast. The usual tendency is for the required kVp value to be over-estimated, since failure to penetrate the object is a more compelling reason for repeating a radiograph than is poor contrast — which might, in fact, be due to other technique faults. Due to the increased radiation intensity at higher kVp values, errors in kVp selection also tend to produce over-exposed radiographs. (These, again, are less likely to lead to 'repeat films' since a high-intensity light source may be used for viewing the darker parts of the image.)

It must be mentioned that some radiographs yield maximum (or sufficient) diagnostic value when contrast is *not* at its highest. Under these circumstances, the term 'optimum kV' fails to have relevance.

Image unsharpness

The intensity of radiation emitted from an X-ray tube increases as the kilovoltage is raised — being approximately proportional to the squared kVp value. Since an X-ray beam generated at a high kilovoltage more easily penetrates an object, there is a further, relative increase in the intensity of the transmitted beam. Additionally, when intensifying screens are used, an increase in kilovoltage tends to raise the intensification factor. The combined result of these effects is that the ability of the X-ray beam to create a radiographic density, increases markedly as the tube kilovoltage is raised. (It is approximately proportional to kVp^4.)

If overexposure is to be avoided when a radiograph is taken at a higher kVp, there must be a compensatory reduction of some other factor. Most usefully, this is a shortening of the exposure time. Thus an increase in the tube kilovoltage, above the basic value required for penetrating the object, can be effective in reducing *movement unsharpness*.

Some illustrations of abdominal radiography may help to explain this point:

To show the outlines of the kidneys (adult patient):
the kilovoltage might typically lie within the range 60–70 kV. The reason would be to maintain the relatively slight difference between the absorption coefficients of renal and perirenal tissue, and record this as radiographic image contrast.

To show a suspected intestinal obstruction:
the kV could be higher than in the previous case. The aim of this examination would be to show (if present) the distended, gas-filled sections of bowel, contrasting with the denser surrounding structures. The contrast inherent in the object is here greater than between a kidney and its surroundings and should be easily visible on a radiograph exposed at 80–90 kV. The increased radiation *intensity* at these higher kilovoltages and its film exposing capability, enable the exposure time (and the accompanying risk of movement unsharpness) to be reduced — a significant point with a patient who is possibly too ill to co-operate fully.

During a fluoroscopic examination, using barium sulphate:
the subject contrast between the opacified stomach or bowel and the surrounding tissues is now so high that the kilovoltage can be raised to 100–130 kV without a significant reduction of radiographic image contrast. The exposure time reduction made possible in this case will help to eliminate *peristaltic* as well as respiratory movement unsharpness.

Radiation protection

When a high kilovoltage is used to generate the X-ray beam (the term 'high' implies being greater than necessary for penetration, and usually indicates a value above 100 kV) less energy tends to be absorbed by the patient from the primary beam. Provided that the reduced image contrast is acceptable, this exposure technique may be used as a means of reducing the dose to the patient. Its benefits are not entirely clear cut, however: the scattered radiation has greater energy and extends further from the volume of tissue irradiated by the primary.

Suggested exercise

— Students should investigate the kilovoltage values used in the X-ray department for the various radiographic projections to establish why, particularly, they are selected.

Related studies

Interactions between X-rays and matter: the influence of changes in beam quality.

24

What determines the required milliampere-seconds value, for any given radiograph?

The milliampere-seconds factor required for a radiograph (i.e., the product of tube current and exposure time) concerns production of a satisfactory *image density*. The milliampere-second is a unit of electrical charge, in which is measured the charge crossing the X-ray tube during an exposure. This value is used to indicate the quantity of X-radiation *produced at the tube target*.

Determination of an mAs value for a radiograph involves factors which

— relate the quantity of radiation *produced at the tube target*, to the quantity *impinging on the image recording system*
— concern the *image-forming efficiency* of the radiation reaching the image recording system.

Reduction of radiation intensity

The radiopacity ('size') of a given object obviously affects attenuation of the X-ray beam passing through to the image recording system. An mAs value is selected to match the object's radiopacity. The other principal factors are:

119

Focus-film distance

Although, strictly, not emitted from a *point* source, the X-ray beam is found to behave approximately according to the inverse square law. Thus the mAs value required for a given image density is directly proportional to the *square of the focus-film distance*.

Secondary radiation grid

Absorption of primary as well as secondary radiation occurs when a grid is used. The effect on image density is expressed by the *grid factor*. This is the factor by which the mAs value has to be multiplied to maintain image density, compared with *not* using a grid.

Tube kilovoltage

Due to its effects on (a) the efficiency of X-ray production at the tube target and (b) the beam's power to penetrate an object, there is an inverse relationship between kV and mAs. When kV is increased, the mAs must be reduced to keep the same quantity of radiation impinging on the image recording system.

Image-forming efficiency

The mAs value for an exposure must take account of the *speed* of the image-recording system: the faster the system, the lower will be the required mAs.

The speed of intensifying screens, as indicated by their intensification factor, is affected by changes in the tube kilovoltage: at higher kV values, the intensification factor tends to increase.

Thus the influence of kV on mAs, mentioned above, is extended when intensifying screens are used. In practice, the image-density-forming power of an X-ray beam (when screens are used) is approximately proportional to kV^4. The mAs values need to be adjusted (inversely) accordingly.

(A well-tried radiographic 'rule of thumb' expresses this relationship by saying that: 'if the kV is increased by 10, the mAs can be halved'. This holds approximately true within the range 50–80 kV.)

Small-field collimation

There are occasions when a large-field radiograph of an object may be followed up by a very much smaller field view of a particular part of the object — e.g., a single vertebra within a region of the spine.

The purpose of collimating the beam closely to the size of this smaller structure is to enhance the contrast, by eliminating the scattered radiation which would otherwise enter the field from surrounding structures (Fig. 15, p. 49).

While excluding the contrast-reducing effect of the scatter, the collimation also reduces the overall image-density-forming effect of the beam.

A restorative increase in mAs needs to be made, in these cases, in proportion to the density lost.

Suggested exercises

— Students should investigate the exposure factors used in the X-ray department, in this instance, to see how the mAs value is adapted to match alterations in (i) focus-film distance; (ii) speed of image recording system; (iii) use of a secondary radiation grid; (iv) beam collimation to a small area; (v) kilovoltage.

25

How does a radiographer decide on the focus-film distance to be used for a projection?

On most occasion, the focus-film distance has already been chosen by previous experience or by well-worn practice. But even so, a radiographer should know *why* a particular distance has proved best — and should be able to make an appropriate amendment if circumstances suggest.

The focus-film distance used for most examinations is approximately 1 metre. This represents a compromise, in that there are arguments both for having a shorter and a greater distance.

In favour of using a shorter distance would be the fact that an X-ray beam's intensity reduces with the square of the distance. Thus it might be argued that at shorter distances there is a tendency for only correspondingly short exposure times to be required. The likelihood that *movement* will cause image unsharpness is thereby reduced.

The use of a larger focus-film distance is mainly argued according to its role in reducing *geometric* unsharpness (Fig. 45), particularly for objects remote from the film.

When the object-film distance is significantly increased, the focus-film distance is, in fact, usually extended (i.e., beyond 1 metre). Two routine examples are the lateral projection of the cervical spine and radiographs of the chest. In both cases, a distance of approximately 1.8 metres is used.

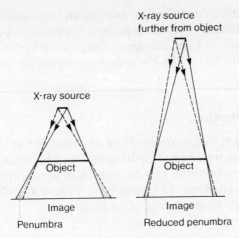

Fig. 45 Reduction in geometric unsharpness: increase of ratio between focus-object distance and object-film distance.

For a lateral projection of the cervical spine, the width of the shoulder separates the object from the film — which must be placed sufficiently low to record the cervico-thoracic area. If the patient's neck is slender (so that a grid is thought unnecessary) and there is adequate immobilisation, the lengthened exposure time implied by the increased distance, is acceptable.

For radiography of the chest, where the air-filled, low density object normally permits very short exposure times, an increased focus-film distance limits geometric unsharpness — even of the fine structures remote from the film (posterior parts on a postero-anterior projection, for example). The increased focus-film distance also minimises magnification of the heart shadow as an aid to diagnosis.

Radiographers can thus adjust the focus-film distances they use, to reduce unsharpness. But two, possibly restricting, influences should be borne in mind:

1. If a focused grid is being used, the focus-film distance must not differ too much from the grid's focused distance. Otherwise 'geometrical cut-off' (absorption of primary) may reduce image density from the side margins of the film, inwards.

2. If the focus-film distance is reduced, there will, in accord-

ance with the inverse square law, be an increase in the intensity of radiation to which a patient is exposed, even though image density is kept constant. Thus, on radiation protection grounds, the focus-film distance must never be 'short'.

Suggested exercise

— Although, in an experimental arrangement, it is difficult to stimulate movement unsharpness (of a phantom), students could make some test exposures to assess the degree to which changes of focus-film distance influence the observed unsharpness of an image.

26

Which causes of image unsharpness are the most important?

One of a radiographer's principal skills lies in being able to:

— recognise *all* the possible causes of unsharpness, in given circumstances
— identify the *likeliest* cause of unsharpness
— reduce the effect of this particular cause, *down to the level of the others*.

Thus, ideally, no single cause should predominate; and the likeliest cause is virtually the 'most important'.

During some radiographic examinations, the likeliest cause of unsharpness will be obvious. For example, when a patient is unconscious and restless, movement is going to present the biggest problem. Under other circumstances the balance between the options will tend to be more subtle.

The choices facing a radiographer may be summarised as follows:

1. If immobilisation is expected to be effective, focal spot size may be minimised and focus-film distance increased to reduce geometric factors; and a 'fine grain' film/screen combination may be employed.

2. If photographic factors are not expected to be obtrusive, a balance must be struck between using a small focal spot (to

minimise penumbra) and maintaining the shortest possible exposure time.

3. If geometric factors are not likely to be dominant (when, for instance, the object is only small and positioned in contact with the film) the likelihood of movement is weighed against the possibility of photographic unsharpness.

Additional points the radiographer may have to consider are:

— the relative importance, on any occasion, of unsharpness and diminished contrast: might the resultant image be clearer if radiation intensity is increased (and exposure time reduced) by raising tube kilovoltage? Will a reduced exposure time be more beneficial than use of a grid?
— concerning radiation protection: in the circumstances, does priority need to be given to reducing the dose to the patient, rather than eliminating (photographic) unsharpness?

Summary

The most important point for students to remember is to maintain an awareness of *all* the possible causes of unsharpness. It would be futile to pursue limitation of one particular cause if, by neglect, others were allowed to be more relevant.

For example, if geometric causes alone are thought to be most important, use of the smallest available focal spot size, with its low mA availability, may lengthen the exposure time to such an extent that movement occurs during the exposure. Even if immobilisation can be secured, it may then be the case that the film/screen combination is incapable of resolving the reduction in penumbra that the smaller focal spot achieves.

An effective aid to radiographers in controlling unsharpness is a reliable knowledge of an X-ray unit's capabilities. These should be established by experiment, using phantoms and all the available image recording systems.

Suggested exercise

— Comparative radiographs of a suitable phantom should be

taken to investigate the actual effects on image unsharpness, of changes in all possible variables.

It is suggested that the radiographs are each given a coded reference letter or number, so that an impartial and uninformed observer can be called in to give an opinion, if necessary.

27

How should an X-ray beam be collimated?

Ideally, the X-ray field should include the whole of the required object but not extend beyond its limits. In this way, the radiation hazard to the object is minimised and the contrast of its image is not unnecessarily reduced. To achieve these requirements, the radiographer must be able to *centre the X-ray beam accurately* to the object and *adjust the field to any appropriate size*.

Variable collimation

The usual piece of equipment enabling these requirements to be met, is the **light-beam collimator** (or **diaphragm**) — Figure 46. This normally provides a rectangular field of any required dimensions.

Students will be familiar with the outward appearance of a light beam collimator. Internally, an angled radiolucent mirror reflects light from a high intensity lamp precisely along the path of X-rays from the tube target. Both light and X-ray beams can then be centred to the object, with the help of markings on the collimator's window; and collimated (restricted) to the required size.

The pairs of collimator leaves ('transverse' and 'longitudinal') can be moved independently but both leaves of each pair are

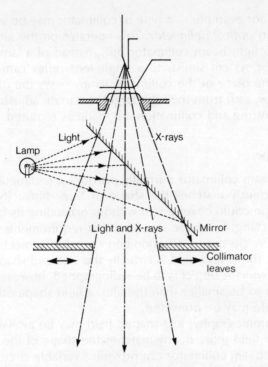

Fig. 46 Light beam collimator: diagram to show principle of operation. Note that the focal spot and the lamp's filament must be equidistant from the mirror.

linked to move symmetrically about the midline.

If there is doubt about the extent of the object, the field can be 'opened up' to *but not beyond* the borders of the film. When a film is not visible to the radiographer, assistance in adjusting field size can be gained from calibrations on the diaphragm movement controls; or from printed guidelines on the collimator window,

The accuracy of a light-beam collimator relies on precise location of the lamp filament and mirror. Should either (usually the mirror) be displaced, X-rays and light will no longer coincide. Fortunately, a simple check radiograph can be taken: with opaque markers indicating the limits of the light field and the X-ray tube's orientation relative to the film. A variation of up to 1 cm at a focus-film distance of 1 m, is usually tolerated.

If a light beam (field) cannot be easily seen — in a brightly-lit room, for example — a type of collimator may be available, termed an *optical delineator*. This operates on the same principle as a light beam collimator but, instead of a lamp, has a viewfinder system similar to a single-lens reflex camera. The eye, in the place of the collimator lamp, views the object via the mirror, as if from the tube target. Accurate adjustments to beam centring and collimation are made as required.

Field shape

A light beam collimator normally provides a rectangular field. This efficiently matches the shape of X-ray films. (No other field shape could cover a film without exceeding its borders.)

The rectangular shape satisfies most requirements: for the routine PA chest and AP abdomen or pelvis projections, for instance, the useful field is virtually the size and shape of the film. If a *specific* object is to be radiographed, however, which is known to be smaller than the film, a field shape other than a rectangle may be preferred.

For mammography, a D-shaped field may be available; and a circular field more nearly matches the shape of the skull.

A light beam collimator can provide a variable circular field, if fitted with lead leaves in the form of an *iris* diaphragm.

Fixed collimators

The main benefit of variable collimation is that any required field size can be produced, *at any focus-film distance*. At standard focus-film distances, however, collimators may be used which have fixed apertures.

Beam collimation on a skull unit, for instance, is commonly provided by using one of a set of plate diaphragms. These give accurate, pre-set fields, shaped to suit particular projections.

Cylindrical cones, once used for beam collimation on all occasions, may still find a use in modern practice. They are more efficient than single plates, at absorbing extra-focal radiation; and may help the radiographer to achieve X-ray beam alignment and field restriction with more confidence, when a light beam cannot easily be projected onto a film.

An example of such an occasion is the taking of intra-oral dental radiographs — in which case, the cone also indicates the focus-film distance.

Some exceptions

As a rule, an X-ray beam must be collimated strictly to the boundaries of the object, in the interests of both radiation protection and image contrast.

An acceptable exception to this, however, occurs when some extremities are radiographed. PA and lateral projections of fingers, for example, may well have their contrast enhanced (subjectively) if the image has a dense surround, to eliminate glare when the radiograph is viewed. It is unlikely that, in such a case, there is an increased radiation hazard to the patient.

Intra-oral dental radiography also raises the suggestion that rules are being broken: the radiation field (possibly circular) is likely to exceed the area of the film being held in the patient's mouth. The reason here is that although confident, accurate beam collimation brings advantages, unwisely speculative restriction of the field can result in an important part of the object being omitted from ('coned-off') the image. The inevitable repeat radiograph then doubles the radiation dose received by the patient.

Occasions when a radiographer cannot see or accurately estimate field size and film position, are very few, however, and with modern equipment beam collimation is usually as easy as it is effective.

Suggested exercises

— Students should examine the various types of beam collimators in use in the X-ray department. Are some more effective than others?
Are some related closely to the design and use (techniques) of the equipment?
— The test for X-ray and light-beam alignment should be carried out under the supervision of a radiographer.

28

Why are contrast agents used?

Conventional image recording systems (X-ray film and intensifying screens) are limited in the degree to which they can record the contrast between component parts of an object. Modern electronic imaging systems have been developed which are sensitive to a much finer degree, to differences between adjacent structures, in their effective atomic numbers and densities. But, since the earliest days of radiography, a solution has been in use which tackles this problem's cause rather than its effect. This is, to change artificially the object's composition, temporarily, to bring its contrast up to a level which film and screens can detect.

TYPES OF CONTRAST AGENT

Contrast agents are divided into two main groupings:

Positive agents

These are substances which have relatively *high effective atomic numbers*. They are chemical compounds containing either barium (atomic number 56) or iodine (atomic number 53). Both are *more radiopaque* than soft tissues of the body (effective atomic numbers 6–7.5).

Barium is used as an aqueous suspension of barium sulphate, and mostly confined to examinations of the alimentary tract. Iodine is used in a variety of forms — mainly in water-soluble organic chemical compounds but also, for a few purposes, in iodised oils.

Negative agents

These are gases: usually carbon dioxide or, simply, air. They contrast with body tissues through having *low densities* and are therefore *radiolucent*.

APPLICATIONS

Contrast agents can be introduced into the body to outline anatomical structures and, in some cases, to add information about physiology. Their uses may be described under two headings.

1. Opacification of body fluids

Iodinated agents are used to make body fluids radiopaque.

Blood

Blood vessels and chambers of the heart are demonstrated following the introduction of a fluid, opaque agent into the blood circulation. Depending on the purpose of the investigation, the variables include:

site of introduction: for example, an artery or a vein — either for a general or selective investigation;
opacity: determined by the concentration of iodine in the compound, usually expressed in milligrams per millilitre.
viscosity and miscibility: these properties determine how readily the agent mixes with and is diluted by the blood, and how easily it can be injected.
volumes used — both per injection and in total.
method of injection: can be directly via a needle or via a catheter fed to a site remote from its insertion. Manual or powered injections can be used, depending on whether

dispersion is preferred or whether the agent is required to enter the blood stream as a collected 'bolus'.

Lymph

Lymph can be opacified, to demonstrate the vessels and nodes, in the technique of lymphography. The contrast agent is introduced via a very fine catheter inserted after minor surgery into a peripheral lymph capillary.

Cerebrospinal fluid

Opacification of cerebrospinal fluid enables the subarachnoid space to be visualised, both around the spinal cord (myelography) and nerve roots (radiculography).

Bile

Bile may be opacified in the following ways:

physiologically, by excretion of a contrast agent from the liver, either slowly following absorption of ingested tablets or powder (cholecystography), or more rapidly following an intravenous injection (i.v. cholangiography), in which case the duct system is shown, as well as the gall bladder;
by direct mixing with an injected agent, following intubation or catheterisation of the common bile duct (operative, post-operative T-tube, or retrograde cholangiography).

Urine

Urine is opacified by excretion from the kidneys of an agent injected intravenously (i.v. urography).

2. Demonstration of cavities (hollow viscera and ducts)

The techniques simply involve mechanical filling — either partial or complete.

Bronchography

The technique of bronchography involves introducing a small

quantity of an iodinated agent into required segments of the bronchial tree, where it adheres to the walls.

Barium techniques

Barium meals and barium enemas also concern demonstration of the walls. But in these cases (unlike bronchi) the structures contract when empty. Distension could be achieved by the sheer volume of liquid which these structures could accommodate but, usually, it is preferred to use a gas. This 'double contrast' technique enables wall lesions to be shown 'face-on' with the minimum of superimposition.

Double contrast

Similar 'double contrast' techniques can be used to demonstrate joint capsules (arthrography) and the urinary bladder (cystography).

Ducts

Duct demonstration is also a type of cavity filling. Such examinations include retrograde filling of the salivary ducts (sialography) and demonstration of the lacrimal apparatus (dacryocystography). For both these techniques a low-viscosity agent is preferred, due to the fine structure of the ducts.

Male urethrography (retrograde) requires a more viscous agent.

Safety

Contrast agents are drugs. As such they must meet stringent safety requirements, including non-toxicity and chemical stability.

Even so, the introduction of a contrast agent into the patient's body is always attended by a risk. For most X-ray examinations, there are accepted contra-indications — i.e., circumstances linked to the patient's condition, under which the examination must not be carried out.

When it is considered safe to go ahead with an examination, the following should be borne in mind:

- Catheterisation, intubation and injection are procedures which can carry risks.
- The use of iodinated agents can precipitate reactions, in a minority of patients. A patient's medical history can sometimes especially alert attention but resuscitation drugs and equipment must always be at hand for use in an emergency.
- The concentration of the agent and the volume used, can be factors determining the patient's safety, particularly when function is seriously impaired.
- The safety of the contrast agent will normally rest upon its being confined to the structure being examined. If, because of an error during its introduction or an unsuspected pathological condition, an agent leaves the required area, complications may develop.

For instance, an injected agent may go outside the vessel for which it is intended (extravasate), and cause irritation or further complications.

If there is a perforation of the alimentary canal, the normally-safe barium sulphate can leak into the mediastinum or peritoneal cavity and cause very serious consequences. (It must be mentioned that clinical suspicion of a perforation is a contra-indication to the use of barium sulphate.)

Summary

Students will see a wide range of contrast agents in use. Procedures are regularly reviewed and revised, as pharmaceutical and radiological research improves the service to patients.

Suggested exercises

— Contrast agents are usually packaged with abundant information about their composition and applications. Students should take advantage of this and other published information, to learn about the agents used in the X-ray department.

— Students must become familiar with the treatment and resuscitation procedures which are initiated, when a patient suffers a reaction to a contrast agent.

Related studies

Contrast agents and their uses.

29

How much contrast is required in a radiographic image?

The answer to this question depends on the circumstances of each exposure.

With too little contrast, a structure may fail to be identified against its surroundings.

On the other hand, the 'object' might be a collection of varying structures among which there is already wide inherent contrast (in terms of their composition). In this case, radiographic enhancement of the contrast could cause loss of detail from both ends of the density range. The image would then, in fact, have too much contrast.

It will be helpful to summarise some of the factors which influence image contrast.

FACTORS WHICH ENHANCE CONTRAST

Contrast agents

Image contrast originates in the object. The use of a contrast agent can increase differences in composition, between a structure and its surroundings.

X-ray tube kilovoltage

The use of a so-called 'optimum' kV will generate X-rays to outline the densest part of the object and maintain a favourable difference in attenuation between its various parts.

Reduction in volume of irradiated tissue

Such a reduction, by collimation of the primary beam and, for abdominal radiography, by compression (displacement), reduces the production of scattered radiation.

Use of a grid

A grid (or, less commonly, an air gap or scatter filter) reduces the amount of scattered radiation (emerging from the object) which reaches the film.

Film/screen combination

Sensitometric response can heighten conversion of the transmitted radiation contrast into eventual image contrast.

FACTORS WHICH CAN BE EMPLOYED TO REDUCE CONTRAST

Included here are only those factors which a radiographer may *positively choose* for the purpose of restricting image contrast.

X-ray tube kilovoltage

The use of a kilovoltage above the 'optimum' value will progressively reduce image contrast.

An increased kV (above the value needed for penetration) is the commonest method used by radiographers to compensate for a wide range of object densities, reducing them to a narrower range of optical densities on a single radiograph.

Examples of the use of a high kilovoltage include a PA projection of the chest to equalise densities of apices and bases; a lateral projection of the thoracic inlet to show the whole course of the airway from the neck, down into the thorax; and radiography of the abdomen after ingestion of barium sulphate.

Other factors

Three minor methods might also be added for completeness. All find their applications when there is an identifiable density (thickness) gradient across a structure.

Graded intensifying screens

A graded screen has a fluorescent layer of increasing thickness, from one end to the other. Thus, it shows a continuous variation in speed: one end is slow, the other is fast.

A pair of graded screens can, for instance, be used for an anteroposterior projection of the thoracic spine, with the slowest area oriented to the upper vertebrae, and the fastest to the lower vertebrae.

Differential beam filtration

A thin, wedge-shaped, aluminium filter is suitable, in some cases, for varying the primary beam intensity across an object's varying density.

An example is a lateral projection of the face, to show skeletal and non-skeletal parts simultaneously.

'Anode heel' effect

A variation can sometimes be detected in the intensity of the primary X-ray beam, along the axis from anode to cathode. Intensity tends to be greater towards the cathode end.

This variation, known as the 'anode heel' effect, can occasionally be used to advantage to offset differences in an object's density.

THE RELATIVE IMPORTANCE OF CONTRAST

While it is usual for a fairly high contrast to be required, its importance should be considered in the broad context of the whole radiographic examination.

There may be occasions when reduction of unsharpness is more important than maintenance of high contrast. In such a case, it may be decided *not* to use a grid, in order to reduce exposure time. If, even without a grid, the exposure time is thought to be too long (with an unco-operating patient, for instance), the tube kilovoltage could be raised to take advantage of the increase in beam intensity and efficiency. The image contrast would fall but the overall diagnostic value of the image might increase.

Radiation protection could, in some cases, take priority over image contrast. Moves, such as omission of a grid, could then be taken.

Summary

The required degree of contrast in a radiographic image is determined by circumstances. It is common for fairly high contrast to be needed to demonstrate a structure which does not differ markedly from its surroundings. On other occasions, lower contrast will be acceptable if it is offset by a reduction in either unsharpness or the radiation hazard to the patient.

In some instances, the high contrast in an object's composition needs to be lessened, in order to record the whole object (or area) on a single radiograph.

A final point: students will be aware that contrast is reduced by use of old or poorly-stored film, and incorrect safelighting or development conditions. These factors should play no part in reducing image contrast, even when low contrast is required. In all circumstances, contrast must be *under control*: reduction must be deliberate and not accidental.

Suggested exercise

— Students could survey some of the techniques used in the X-ray department, to see how importantly image contrast is regarded — and which manoeuvres are used to achieve the various results.

30

Why are X-rays regarded as dangerous?

When living tissue is exposed to an X-ray beam, it absorbs energy. Ionisation occurs which initiates chemical and physical reactions. These can lead to biological changes. Some of the changes are reversible but some are not — and it is considered that there is no lower limit to the radiation dose which may cause harmful biological effects.

Biological damage may be classified under either of two headings:

somatic — i.e., affecting the cells of the patient's body. Such damage will occur in parts of the body which receive radiation directly but may subsequently spread elsewhere if, for example, blood-forming tissue is affected.

genetic — i.e., being revealed only in a future generation. Such effects will follow mutation or chromosomal changes in gonadal germ cells (ova or spermatazoa).

An alternative grouping of biological effects, could be into:

immediate — those which are seen relatively soon after exposure (within days) such as a reddening of the skin ('erythema') in the exposed area.

long-term — i.e., becoming apparent only years after the exposure such as malignant changes in cell growth.

Acute, rapidly evident effects of an X-ray exposure are unlikely to occur following the radiation doses normally received by patients during diagnostic radiography.

Long-term effects, however, can result from diagnostic X-ray exposure. The risks of these are considered to increase in proportion to the quantity of radiation and the volume of tissue exposed. It is thus essential for radiographers to minimise the number and magnitude of exposures and to restrict irradiated volumes whenever possible.

Related studies

Students should see available reports of surveys into the uses and effects radiation, and an introductory text on radiobiology.

31

How do radiographers protect themselves against X-radiation?

Early 'pioneer' radiation workers had only primitive equipment and incomplete knowledge of the harm which can result from X-ray exposure. They suffered injuries and, in some awful instances, died as a direct result of their occupation.

Set against this background, it is easy for a modern radiographer to be complacent: up-to-date equipment with remote control, fast imaging systems and elaborate protection devices have made radiography a very safe profession. But safety depends on the operator's care in observing and exercising the rules and regulations.

The first step for a student to take is to learn the regulations governing the safe use of X-rays. There are national safety requirements covering equipment and procedures; and local rules which apply the general regulations to individual X-ray departments. Students will be required to learn the local rules in every X-ray department which they attend during their training, and sign a statment to confirm this.

The hazard of scattered radiation

It will be assumed as understood that a radiographer must **never** allow himself or herself, or any colleague, to be exposed to the primary X-ray beam, when a patient is being radiographed.

But scattered radiation, although limited by beam collimation and all other procedures to protect the patient, has also to be considered.

The protective screen or cubicle surrounding the control panel of an X-ray generator provides protection under normal circumstances. During fluoroscopy, however, or use of X-rays in an operating theatre or hospital ward, a radiographer might not be able to go or remain behind such a screen. On these occasions, a protective apron must be worn and use made of other absorbing barriers, as well as distance from the radiation source. It is also the radiographer's responsibility in these circumstances to advise other, non-radiographic staff about the need for safety precautions when the X-ray tube is energised.

On rare occasions, it may be necessary for a patient to be held or closely attended during an X-ray exposure. Being a person who is occupationally at risk, a radiographer must not carry out such a task. Instead, a relative or friend of the patient should be invited to assist. This person must be equipped as fully as possible with protective clothing and positioned outside the primary beam.

Personal monitoring

As a safety precaution, every student and member of staff in an X-ray department will, whilst on duty, wear a radiation monitoring device. This is normally either a thermoluminescent sachet or a photographic film. Its purpose is to detect and measure any accidental radiation to which its wearer is exposed. The remoteness of the possibility of such a dose, must not make staff careless about wearing monitoring devices at all times, in the correct position, reporting any loss immediately and exchanging old for new promptly at the end of every monitoring period.

Mutual responsibilities

As well as needing to protect themselves, for their own and

their families' sakes, radiographers need to exercise a responsibility for the safety of their colleagues.

The door of a radiographic room, carelessly left open while a patient is being radiographed, not only constitutes a lack of respect for the patient's privacy, it presents a radiation hazard to staff outside the room.

Hazard warning lights and notices at the entrances to radiographic rooms must be clearly sited and always respected.

A common responsibility can also be exercised by drawing to the attention of the Radiation Safety Officer in an X-ray department, deficiencies in room design and layout. The most carefully laid plans can prove to contain errors and omissions, when put into practice. Suggested improvements will always be considered in the interests of safety.

Related studies

Regulations, both national and local, concerning the safe use of X-rays. Design features of radiographic rooms, including siting of equipment and doors, and provision of protective barriers. Personnel monitoring.

32

Why is identification of a radiograph so important?

A radiograph is a medical document. As such, it must bear sufficient information to identify clearly:

— the patient
— the date of the examination
— other anatomical and technical data which are necessary for a correct interpretation of the image.

Radiographers are responsible for ensuring that this information is recorded permanently on every radiograph.

The consequences of not attending to this responsibility could be very serious. The absence of the patient's name from a radiograph could necessitate a repeat examination — with the accompanying extra hazards and expense. The marking of the *wrong* name on a radiograph could have even more serious consequences, particularly if *two* patients having similar examinations were somehow to get their names interchanged. If undetected, such an error could lead to either or both of the patients receiving incorrect, and perhaps irreversible, medical treatment.

The importance of recording the date (and in some cases, the time) of the examination is obvious if the patient is already into a programme of medical treatment: the sequence of radiographs should show precisely the course of the patient's

147

response to treatment. Any radiograph, however — even if seeming to be a 'one-off', unrelated to other examinations — must bear the date of its exposure. Subsequent development of the patient's condition may create an importance for this date which cannot, originally, be anticipated.

Methods

The only satisfactory, permanent methods of recording the patient's name and the date on a radiograph are those which use the X-ray film's photographic sensitivity.

All these methods require that a small, measured area of the film is protected against X-ray exposure when the patient is radiographed. This is achieved by the use of a thin rectangular lead block fixed into the front of every cassette. The identification area slightly reduces the space available for the radiographic image but, since it is located at the edge of the film, interference is usually avoided. It is necessary, however, that the radiographer is aware of the location of the identification area so that, by orientation of the cassette, it can be kept away from any critical feature of the radiographic image.

The identification equipment exposes the film in this area, to light either from an electric lamp, reflected from an identifying card or transmitted through a stencil; or from an activated, luminescent identification card.

Older types of equipment could only be used under darkroom safelighting conditions because the film had to be unloaded from its cassette. This normally meant that the radiographer — rather than be absent from the work in the radiographic room — had to delegate the task of identifying the radiographs to a darkroom technician. Such delegation did not, however, apply to the *responsibility* for correct identification and, in practice, there could be difficulties.

Newer 'daylight' equipment has brought to radiographers the opportunity for personally identifying their radiographs, accurately, immediately and permanently.

Some technical information can be added to the patient's name and the date, within the identification area on a radiograph. Alternatively, opaque letters or numerals can be affixed to the front of the cassette (or film holder) to record necessary data. Examples include:

— anatomical markers
— confirmation of the patient's position (supine, erect, prone)
— timing of the exposure — e.g. post-injection during an intravenous urogram
— phase of respiration or other activity, at the time of the exposure
— tomographic pivot height.

Suggested exercise

— Students should investigate the methods currently in use for identifying radiographs (Name/Date and other data) in their X-ray departments. If more than one system is used, which gives the most reliable results? If a new system has been introduced recently, in what ways is it more efficient than the former system?

33

How are anatomical markers used?

There is an accepted system of marking radiographs with which student radiographers must become conversant.

Anteroposterior and postero-anterior projections

Conventionally, both AP and PA radiographs are viewed 'from the front' — as if the patient is in the anatomical position, facing the person who is viewing the radiograph. The patient's left-hand side is then on the viewer's right.

The skeleton, however — part of which appears on most radiographs — is symmetrical about the median plane (left mirroring right). Thus, since a radiograph is translucent, there is a risk that it might be viewed wrongly — i.e., from the reverse side, with the right and left sides being mistaken for each other. Even the single organs within the thorax and abdomen cannot be accepted as reliable indicators of right and left sides.

To avoid such confusion, some indication of the patient's left or right side is always marked on a radiograph. This usually takes the form of a small opaque letter 'R' or 'L', placed near the edge of the film.

An anatomical marker is applied to a film so that it can be read correctly by a person viewing the radiograph convention-

150

ally. Thus the patient's right-hand side is identified by a letter 'R' on an AP radiograph, but on a PA projection it is marked, from the X-ray tube's aspect, with an 'Я'.

AP and PA radiographs of the head, neck and trunk are marked in order to distinguish left side from right side. Radiographs of limbs — even if they only show one side of the body — must also be marked, to confirm that side, as distinct from the opposite.

Lateral projections

Although, in the case of the head, neck and trunk, *both* sides are shown superimposed on a lateral projection, the radiograph is marked to indicate *the side nearer the film* — which, by its position, will be shown with less unsharpness than the side remote from the film.

There is, however, no conventionally 'correct' system of viewing lateral projections; markers may therefore be placed either 'AP' or 'PA'.

(In some X-ray departments, the method of viewing lateral projections of the skull, neck and trunk, is as if patients are being examined by fluoroscopy, with the side under examination nearer the image intensifier input screen. According to this method, the patient 'faces' the observer's left for left laterals, and the right for right laterals. Markers are therefore placed 'PA'.)

Lateral projections of extremities are simply marked with an 'R' or an 'L' to indicate which side of the body has been radiographed.

Oblique projections

AP Oblique and PA Oblique projections are marked and viewed in the same manner as the basic AP and PA projections. Lateral Oblique projections are treated as basic Lateral projections.

A supplementary system is used by some radiographers when comparable pairs of oblique projections are taken of right and left paired structures: the oblique projection which specifically shows the right-hand structure is marked with an 'R' (only) and the complementary oblique is marked with an 'L' (only).

Further points

1. It is common for two or more projections of an extremity to be recorded side by side, together on a single film. In these cases, only one projection (per film) need be marked.

2. If matching projections of both extremities are recorded together on a single film it is a common precaution to make this clear by including both right and left markers on the film.

3. Special 'code' markings are in use within X-ray departments for identifying mammographic and intra-oral dental radiographs.

Suggested exercise

— Students should find out which particular methods are in use in the X-ray department, for anatomical marking of radiographs.

34

Why do some patients need to be specially prepared for their X-ray examinations?

Students will have seen that all patients need some form of preparation, however elementary, before being radiographed.

Physical preparation may simply involve removal of clothing which, perhaps because of its thickness or metallic fasteners, would superimpose a shadow on the radiograph. Similarly, if they would interfere with the image, dentures, glasses and other opaque accessories are removed.

Mental preparation — at its simplest level, a brief outline of the procedure, before it begins — is a courtesy to the patient and, if active co-operation is required, may have a bearing on the examination's success.

For some X-ray examinations, however, patients need more preparation than can be carried out during the few minutes before they are radiographed. The following examples illustrate this.

1. Examination of the alimentary canal requires that the part being examined is as empty as can be achieved. Otherwise, residual material will interfere with the demonstration — either by blocking the lumen, to prevent passage of the contrast agent; or by creating 'filling defects' which mimic or conceal pathological conditions.

Thus, before a barium meal examination, the patient's

stomach must be empty. This is usually achieved by denying the patient food and drink for 6–8 hours beforehand.

For a clear examination of the large bowel by a barium enema, dietary restrictions ('low residue' rather than total fasting) must be adopted 2–3 days beforehand, and any tendency to constipation counteracted by use of laxatives. A few hours before the examination, it is usual for the patient to have a colonic washout.

2. Clearance from the bowels of both heavy faecal matter and excess gas, is also a routine preparation for abdominal X-ray examinations of structures other than the alimentary canal. The renal tract, abdominal blood vessels and lymph vessels and the biliary tract are all, to some extent, visualised 'through' the alimentary canal. The less it superimposes a pattern on the image, in these cases, therefore, the clearer will be their demonstration.

3. More particular management of the patient's diet may be required for examinations of the biliary tract, where preliminary use of or abstinence from fatty foods and the degree of hydration, can be important.

4. When a patient is diabetic, dietary preparation, with adjustment of insulin dosage, requires very careful management.

5. The technique of bronchography requires preparation of the patient by a physiotherapist, to supervise postural drainage — i.e., removal of bronchial secretions by means of gravity. This, again, is an emptying procedure, to ensure efficient use of the contrast agent.

6. X-ray investigations of the cardiovascular and central nervous systems may require premedication or sedation of the patient. If a general anaesthetic is to be administered, the full preparation for this must be undertaken.

Mental preparation of the patient increases in importance, in proportion to the complexity of the X-ray examination. This responsibility may, to some extent, be shared with ward nursing and medical staff, since patients often need to be admitted to the hospital beforehand. The radiographer's responsibility still remains, however, for confirming and adding to the information supplied to the patient.

Suggested exercise

— An X-ray department usually has a stock of printed instruction sheets for patients and/or ward staff, regarding preparation for X-ray examinations. Students should collect examples of these, and familiarise themselves with the procedures.

35

Why are a patient's previous radiographs so important?

Students will have noticed that, before any patient undergoes an X-ray examination, checks are made with the patient and the referring clinician, about previous radiographs. These checks should be as exhaustive as possible, in the circumstances, and include the possibility of radiographs' having been taken at other hospitals.

It may be important for the radiographer to have the opportunity to see a patient's previous radiographs:

— when planning which projections are to be taken, to show the required part of the patient most clearly
— when positioning the patient: an unusually sited or extensive structure or lesion, not obvious outwardly, can indicate the need for modification to routine procedures
— when selecting exposure factors: a pathological condition, for instance, which alters the radiopacity of a structure or area, can be disclosed by previous radiographs.

The overall benefits of these points include a possible reduction in the radiation hazard for the patient, and time-saving for both patient and radiographer.

A further benefit to the patient will arise if the radiological report on the examination is more comprehensive, by reason

156

of the radiologist's being able to comment on the patient's condition in relation to a previous occasion.

Suggested exercise

— Students should become familiar with the usual routes along which investigations can be made about previous radiographs, if a patient arrives for an examination without this having been checked. An understanding of the filing systems for radiographs, request cards and reports will be necessary.

36

How do radiographers protect their patients against X-radiation?

Almost every aspect of a radiographer's work has a bearing on the radiation hazards to which patients are subjected. The following sequence identifies some of these points.

1. Operation of equipment

Radiographers will be fully conversant with the procedures for safe operation of their equipment. But periodic checks should be made that the equipment remains in sound working order.

2. Checking of requests

Checking the validity of each request for an X-ray examination (i.e., that it has been made by an appropriate medical or dental officer) is the first step.

Interpretation of the request is then required. In some cases, a radiographer may need to ask a senior colleague or radiologist, or refer to the requesting clinician, or even ask the patient for supplementary information before deciding on the programme of radiographs that need to be taken.

3. Reception of the patient

Firstly, the patient must be identified. Then, if some form of preparation for the examination is supposed to have been carried out, a check is made on this. Incorrect preparation must not remain undiscovered until the patient has already received an X-ray exposure.

A further check may then be made, if the patient is female and of 'child-bearing age' and due to have an X-ray examination of the abdomen or pelvis: she must confirm that she is not pregnant. This is a check, in the sense that the clinician requesting the X-ray examination should already have confirmed this point, but it is a radiographer's duty to reinforce this.

The reason for this precaution is that an embryo or fetus is particularly susceptible to the biological damage which might ensue from exposure to X-rays — especially when it is likely to received a 'whole body' exposure. Discussion of her possible pregnancy, with a patient, must naturally be conducted with privacy and discretion. The main risk of an error, in this matter, will arise when a woman has so recently conceived that she is unaware of her early pregnancy — i.e., cesssation of menstruation has yet to become evident.

If there is no urgency about carrying out the X-ray examination, it is usual practice to observe the radiation protection 'Ten-Day Rule'. This involves postponing the X-ray examination until after the onset of the patient's next menstrual period and requesting that she should attend for X-ray examination some time during the ten days from this date. Ovulation normally occurs on the 14th day: thus it can be virtually guaranteed that the patient is not pregnant during this ten-day span.

Checking the possibility of an early pregnancy should be a routine measure when an X-ray examination is requested and, again, when an appointment is made. But it must be mentioned that the Ten-Day Rule is waived in some cases. Patients who are medically incapable of conceiving are exempted, as are nuns.

Exemption is also exercised in cases where the need for an X-ray examination is urgent. The diagnostic use of X-rays is requested by a clinician after consideration of the so-called 'Benefit-Risk Relationship'. This expresses the fact that the benefit of a radiological report on the patient's condition (with its subsequent implications for successful treatment and recovery) has to be weighed against the risk of biological harm which may result from exposure to X-rays.

This decision must be considered when *any* X-ray examination is requested — and the radiographer's skilled technique should confirm the clinician's judgement that the benefit outweighs the risk.

A full explanation of the procedure is given to the patient, before it begins.

4. Radiographic techniques

The aim, throughout an examination, is to gain an appropriately large amount of diagnostic information, while exposing the patient to a minimum amount of radiation.

Absolute points include careful positioning, centring, X-ray beam collimation, use of gonad shields and other protective masking and use of automatic exposure timing equipment.

Balanced against their effects on image quality are the use of fast image recording materials, possible exclusion of a grid, and kilovoltage selection.

Responsible precautions include taking advantage of information that previous radiographs may provide and, for future use, recording exposure factors and other data on the patient's card.

A performance marked by the skill which experience brings includes systematic care that every step of the procedure goes according to plan, with every possible problem foreseen, if not expected. Such points need not be complicated; they include simply positioning patients comfortably and in such a way that they remain fully in the radiographer's line of vision throughout. (A patient who is even slightly uncomfortable may take the opportunity for self re-positioning, when the radiographer retreats behind the screen!)

5. Special circumstances

It is often said that, in the interest of radiation protection, 'special care' is taken when radiographing certain patients. A statement as simple as this can be misleading — particularly to students. It is invidious to suggest that special care is offered to certain patients if, by implication, others might receive less. The true position is one of sensible emphasis on particularly relevant aspects. No neglect is implied to the overall care of any patient. The following examples are offered as illustrations.

a. When radiographs are taken of patients who can be considered to have 'reproductive capacity' (an unlikeable expression, but succinct), care must be taken to prevent or reduce radiation exposure of the gonads.

Geriatric patients are not put at extra risk by omission of this precaution. Indeed, many would be amused by its inclusion.

b. Immobilisation aids are considered as part of radiation protection, in that they may reduce the need for a radiograph to be repeated. Their use is particularly recommended when radiographing infants and young children because these patients experience more fear and understand the need to keep still, much less than adults.

c. While it is recommended that radiographers should make a record of the exposure factors used for each patient, there are some instances (anatomical parts which have negligible variation in size, from patient to patient; and when exposures are automatically timed) where this practice is of only token importance.

A record *is* important, however, when follow-up radiographs are expected, at intervals in the future. The progress of a patient's lung condition is an example, particularly if the radiographs are exposed in a ward rather than the X-ray department — and would, in such a case, include a record of focus-film distance, and type of intensifying screens, as well as kV and mAs.

d. The programme of projections taken during any radiographic procedure, can be varied (either by reduction or increase) to match individual patient's needs. Such variations (an aspect of the Benefit/Risk relationship) would normally be made after discussion between radiographer and radiologist. A decision would include consideration of the extra or reduced radiation, in the context of the whole, and the radiation sensitivity of the tissues being exposed.

Thus, a supplementary projection of an extremity would be sanctioned more readily than an extra radiograph of the abdomen, during an intravenous urogram. In the latter case, since exposure to the gonads and blood-forming tissue in the pelvis and spine is involved, the tendency would be to reduce the number of exposures.

Suggested exercises

Students should look for examples within their departments, of alternative imaging techniques not involving the use of X-rays — notably ultrasound and, possibly, nuclear magnetic resonance (zeugmatography).

— Were or are these techniques introduced to remove the hazards of tissue ionisation?

Related studies

Radiation protection regulations including the Ten-Day Rule and its implementation.

37

What is a 'control' radiograph?

Radiographic appearances are potentially misleading. Distortion and superimposition occur and patients can have structural and functional variations from 'normal'. A control is a standard against which observations can be checked and validated.

'Both sides for comparison' is a phrase commonly used when some radiographic techniques are being described. The principle employed in these cases is that a radiograph of the supposed 'normal' structure (uninjured or assumed not to be affected by disease) will be of value in interpreting the appearance of the (suspected) abnormal.

Applications of this principle include examinations of the sacro-iliac and sternoclavicular joints and optic foramina; radiographs of children, to investigate bony pathology or trauma in regions of developing bone (epiphyses); and demonstration of ligamentous damage to some joints, where 'stressed' and 'unstressed' appearances can be compared.

A fracture of the femoral neck tends to cause external rotation of the limb. On an anteroposterior radiograph, the effect of external rotation is foreshortening, which can make interpretation difficult. Corrective internal rotation to restore an ideal relationship between object and X-ray beam is contraindicated by the injury. But a comparable foreshortened view of the unaffected femoral neck, with that leg also externally rotated, can be taken to help distinguish between abnormal and normal.

More common than any of these examples are routine antero-posterior and postero-anterior projections of the skull, thorax and abdomen, taken with the X-ray beam directed along the median plane. If careful radiographic technique produces a symmetrical appearance, right and left act as complementary controls for each other.

Another common usage of the term 'control' is in describing preliminary radiographs taken before an examination involving a contrast agent. Radiologically, a control, in this sense (to show the abdomen before intravenous urography, for instance) will demonstrate calculi and other opacities which might later be concealed by the introduced contrast agent. The technique of subtraction employs a similar principle.

Control radiographs taken before contrast agent examin-ations, also provide information about:

— exposure factor selection
— positioning of the patient
— centring and collimation of the X-ray beam
— preparation of the patient: the presence of undue amounts of faecal matter or gas, or even residual barium sulphate, can enable an examination to be terminated before time, money and radiation are needlessly wasted.

38

What 'functional states' may radiographs be required to show?

Some structures have radiographic appearances which are independent of their orientation. A postero-anterior projection of the hand, for example, will appear the same whether the hand is pronated, as is usual, or positioned against a vertical film and radiographed with a horizontal X-ray beam.

In contrast, the radiographic appearance of a patient's chest is not independent of the circumstances of its exposure. The standard PA projection of a chest shows how it responds (i) to gravity, with the patient erect, and (ii) to full inspiration.

Response to inspiration and expiration is not confined to thoracic organs. Structures in the upper abdomen also respond to diaphragmatic movements. Respiratory manoeuvres can be used to elucidate ambiguous appearances — to identify opacities, for example.

The force of gravity exerts a particular effect on any structure which is mobile. Fluid and gas respond most readily. Students may be familiar with comparative 'supine' and 'erect' appearances of the abdomen, and other differences which the patient's particular position can make to the appearance of otherwise identical projections.

The state of responding to pressure from body weight can be shown by radiographs, taken with the patient erect, of the vertebral column, knee joints, and arches of the foot. Radiographs can also show the spine's functional response to flexion and extension.

The introduction of contrast agents enables many organ functions to be demonstrated, mostly with the aid of fluoroscopic techniques. Those which usually involve radiographs alone, include intravenous urography, showing the excretory function of the kidneys, and examinations of biliary tract function.

In order to carry out such examinations particularly, students must learn thoroughly the relevant facts of function and physiology, as well as anatomy.

39

How significant is image magnification?

All radiographic images are larger than the objects they repre-
sent. This is due to the divergent nature of the X-ray beam and
the separation between object and image planes. The magnification factor — i.e., the ratio between image and object
sizes — is determined by the ratio between the focus-film distance and the focus-object distance (Fig. 47).

Magnification is not normally detrimental to a radiographic
image; it may, in fact, improve visibility of detail. The technique of macroradiography is used to create a considerably
magnified image, for this purpose.

Unfortunately, geometric unsharpness (with which magnification is sometimes wrongly confused) has to be borne in
mind. The link lies in the common effect of an increase in
object-film distance: this makes *both* magnification *and*
geometric unsharpness greater.

If the true dimensions of an object need to be measured, as
in the technique of pelvimetry, this can be achieved by (i)
equalising magnification across the whole of the object, and
(ii) measuring the distances which control the magnification
factor.

Magnification may be significant if it is unequal in different
parts of an image: this causes distortion.

167

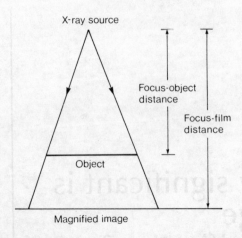

Fig. 47 Image magnification: factor determined by ratio between focus-film distance and focus-object distance.

Two techniques concerned with magnification are now briefly described.

Macroradiography

This is a technique in which image magnification is deliberately increased, despite the fact of an accompanying enlargement of geometric unsharpness. Its advantage over optical magnification of an 'ordinary size' radiograph lies in the absence of enlarged (more conspicuous) photographic grain — and unsharpness.

The principle is simple; the ratio — focus-film distance: focus-object distance — is increased to equal the desired magnification factor. This increase is achieved by (compared with ordinary radiography) widening the separation between object and film. (A reduction in the focus-object distance would increase the radiation hazard to the patient, and reduce the available field size.)

The problem of geometric unsharpness is solved by the use of an ultra-fine focal spot; 0.3 mm or less. This unfortunately, creates a further problem: the low rating of such a small focus inevitably lengthens exposure times — which, with a greater focus-film distance, are increased already. Fortunately the air gap between object and film makes use of a grid unnecessary but, even so, immobilisation of the object is very important.

Pelvimetry

This obstetric technique is a means of measuring with accuracy required diameters of the maternal pelvis. The changes in management of pregnancy which diagnostic ultrasound have brought about, have made this technique less common than formerly. Accordingly, the following account is intended to convey only the principle underlying the commonest pelvimetric projection: the lateral.

The technique involves three stages:

1. The required diameters are positioned parallel to the film. For measuring anteroposterior diameters of the pelvic canal, a lateral projection is used.

2. The measurements affecting magnification are recorded while the patient is positioned for the projection. The focus-object distance is found by subtraction of the object film distance from the focus-film distance. (The object, in this case, is the patient's median plane.)

3. All direct measurements from the radiograph are reduced by (inverted) application of the magnification factor.

Suggested exercise

— An experimental macroradiograph of a phantom should be taken. The magnification factor should be calculated and used as a check between the measurements (a) read from the radiograph and (b) taken of the phantom.

Related studies

Practical techniques of macroradiography and pelvimetry (if these can be observed by the student).

40

What is tomography?

This term means radiography of a *slice* or *layer* through the object rather than of its whole. There are two clearly distinguishable techniques, both described as 'tomography'.

Computed tomography is a technique which involves collecting information about the structure and composition of a slice through the object and then, by means of a computer, analysing and assembling the information as an image of this slice. The tomographic character of such images is not their only important feature: the X-ray detector system used is very much more sensitive than photographic film, to variations in X-ray intensity. The images thus reveal tissue differences beyond the capability of conventional radiography. This and other imaging techniques which employ computer processing, lie outside the scope of this introductory text.

Conventional tomography is practised using a conventional X-ray tube and image recording system (film and intensifying screens) although under this broad heading there are several variables.

CONVENTIONAL TOMOGRAPHY

Principle

Separation of the image of any required layer, from all other parts of the object, is achieved by movement. With reference to Figure 48: X-ray tube and film are linked mechanically, so that both move about a common pivot (fulcrum).

Movement of the X-ray tube from 1 to 2, causes the shadow of the patient's body to move in the opposite direction (also shown as 1 to 2, as the film travel). But within this composite shadow are *separate shadows* of planes through the body, each moving at a different speed. Only the shadow of a plane parallel to the film, passing through the pivot, moves at the speed of the film. Thus, a sharp image of this plane is recorded.

Planes above the pivot (such as A, in Fig. 48) cast shadows which move faster than the film. The shadows of planes below the pivot (such as C) move more slowly than the film. All these, therefore, move in relation to the film and record blurred images.

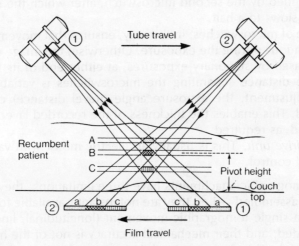

Fig. 48 The principle of tomography. During the exposure (1–2) only structures along the pivot plane (B) move at the same speed as the film. Those above (A) and below (C) move at a different speed and produce blurred images. Note that the shaded areas are representative of the whole planes, and not just localised parts.

Equipment

The simplest form of tomographic equipment is an attachment for use with a conventionally mounted (separate) X-ray tube and couch. It has three parts:

A connecting rod which links the X-ray tube mount (axis of rotation at level of tube target) to the bucky/cassette assembly (axis of rotation at the level of the film) via the tomography pivot. If, as in this arrangement, tube and film move in parallel planes, the focus-film distance changes during the exposure. The connecting rod thus needs to be variable in length.

A pivot unit. This is rigidly fixed to a side rail on the couch. An adjustment device allows the pivot to be moved up or down to required heights above the couch top, measured on an adjacent scale.

Two microswitches on the pivot unit, operated by pressure from the connecting rod, start and end the tomographic exposure. The usual 'exposure' switch on the control panel initiates movement of the tube and film. The tomographic exposure begins when the connecting rod reaches the first microswitch. It is ended by the second microswitch, after which the movement slows to a halt.

Use of microswitches, in this way, ensures that movement is continuous during the exposure. Otherwise, the image would be biased by stationary exposures, at either end of its travel.

The distance separating the microswitches is variable. By its adjustment, the exposure angle (travel distance) can be varied. This enables the thickness of the recorded layer to be altered, as required.

A drive unit. This is usually an electric motor with variable speed control.

Tomographic attachments have three limitations: they need to be assembled — i.e., they are not instantly available for use; only a single tomographic movement (longitudinal, linear) is provided; and their mechanical accuracy is not of the highest standard. This is aggravated by repeated connection and disconnection, and reduces image quality.

These deficiencies are remedied (although at a price) by use of equipment specially designed and built for tomography. This instantly provides refined, accurate facilities.

Technique

To a patient lying (it seems) within noisy, gyrating X-ray equipment, a tomographic examination can be a frightening experience. An explanation and 'demonstration run' by the radiographer are probably essential to satisfactory conduct of the examination.

Tomography will be requested to provide information about a specific structure or lesion. The radiographer needs to centre the X-ray beam accurately to this point, longitudinally and transversely as for an ordinary radiography. For this, the X-ray beam must be in a 'neutral' position, at right angles to the film. Additionally, the pivot height needs to be adjusted to the appropriate level.

These centring procedures cannot be carried out without reference to the patient's most recent plain radiographs. If more recent pathological changes are thought possibly to have occurred, the tomographic examination must be preceded by taking plain radiographs. Two projections, mutually at right angles are required. Measurements taken from these (with due regard for the magnification they show) will provide the necessary guidance.

If an appropriate radiograph is not available to give a guide to pivot height (for an abdominal structure, for instance) an approximate setting must be made, using previous experience of similar examinations.

When all the technical factors have been selected, the tomographic examination can then proceed.

Suggested exercise

— Students should thoroughly inspect the tomographic equipment used in the X-ray department, seeing how its construction provides the facilities required by the tomographic principles.

Related studies

Tomographic equipment and techniques.

41

What factors does a radiographer control during conventional tomography?

Centring

As with ordinary radiography, the X-ray beam needs to be centred to the required structure. But tomography brings an additional dimension to centring: not only is longitudinal and transverse adjustment needed, the height of the pivot must be set centrally to the area of interest. Reliably recent radiographs (two projections, mutually at right angles) are usually needed for this; otherwise, the pivot height is set approximately, using previous experience of similar examinations.

Exposure factors

Exposure factors need to be set: tube kilovoltage and (unless automatic exposure control is available) milliampere-seconds to correspond to the film/screen combination being used. (The focus-film distance is probably already fixed and a standard grid used.)

Tomographic exposures are usually switched on and off by microswitches activated by the connecting rod between tube and film, during its movement. Thus exposure times are determined by the length of the path travelled by the tube (or film) during the exposure, and the speed of travel. Of these two factors, the more important is the length of the travel path. If this is altered, to change the nature of the tomographic image, compensatory adjustment must be made to either the speed of travel or the tube current (mA).

The normal exposure timer on the control panel remains in circuit during tomography and determines the action (intervention) of the tube overload prevention circuit. It is set to a time which just exceeds the tomographic (movement-switched) exposure time, in readiness to operate if the exposure-terminating microswitch fails. If set for too short a time, it will end the tomographic exposure prematurely to produce an asymmetric travel pattern.

Pattern of tube/film travel

The image blurring of structures away from the pivot plane, depends on the pattern of tube/film movement. As they are superimposed on the required (pivot plane) image, it is important that the other, so-called, 'redundant shadows' are spread across the radiograph to interfere with the image as little as possible. Specialised tomographic equipment offers a range of movements (including linear, circular, elliptical, spiral and hypocycloidal) from which a radiographer can select to suit the anatomical configuration of the object. Ideally, the redundant shadows should spread in such a manner as to be unrecognisable. The complicated movement patterns are efficient in this respect. Simple movements offer the advantage, however, of being completed within a short exposure time — an important point, when immobilisation is likely to be difficult.

Thickness of the recorded layer ('cut')

Tomography is, technically, a very interesting technique. But it has a subjective aspect which can frustrate a student's attempts to identify absolute rules and relationships.

For example, it must be accepted that a slight degree of unsharpness does not make an image unrecognisable. Moreover, the extent to which a degree of unsharpness confuses a viewer, depends on that person's individual ability to recognise the features of the image, despite the unsharpness.

The sharply-recorded layer of a tomograph is, in theory, as thin as the axis about which tube and film are moved. In practice, however, the *slight* unsharpness associated with structures lying adjacent to this layer, is insufficient to make them *un*recognisable. They thus increase the observed layer thickness.

The boundaries of the 'sharp' layer (although hard to define) can, however, be moved nearer to or further from the pivot, under given circumstances, by variations of the geometry of tube/film movement.

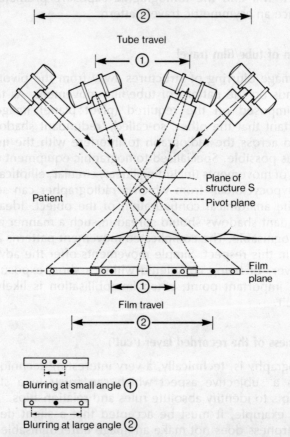

Fig. 49 Tomography: influence of tube travel distance (exposure angle) on thickness of recorded plane (cut). An increase in the travel distance (angle) creates more blurring of structures remote from the pivot plane. The recorded plane thickness (tomographic cut) is thus reduced.

Figure 49 shows a structure, S, positioned away from the pivot plane. (To simplify this description, linear tomographic movement is assumed.) The small exposure angle (travel distance 1) creates a difference between movement of the film and of the shadow of S. If, despite this difference, the image of S is at the limit of being recognised, its distance from the pivot represents half of the 'cut' thickness.

Use of the large exposure angle (travel distance 2) increases the movement differences between the film and the shadow of S, and takes the image of S beyond the boundary of being recognisable. In other words, it reduces the thickness of the 'cut', since the structure whose image now lies on the boundary between 'sharp' and (too) 'unsharp' will be found closer to the pivot plane.

Thus, the thickness of the sharply-recorded tomographic layer is inversely related to the distance travelled by the X-ray tube (or film) during the exposure. Since this relationship implies a fixed vertical distance between tube and film, it is more absolutely accurate to refer to an exposure angle. With linear and circular movements expression of an angle is certainly more simple. Narrow-angle tomography to show wide 'zones' rather than thin slices, is termed **zonography**.

Note, however, that for a given exposure angle, the distance moved for a circular movement is approximately three times greater than for a linear movement (πd, compared with d). It might be expected, therefore, that the thickness of cut is reduced to one third, by a change from linear to circular movement. In practice, this relationship may be modified by other factors.

A radiographer's decision to reduce or increase the 'thickness of cut' will be influenced by:

The thickness of the structure to be tomographed. For small structures, such as the auditory ossicles, only very thin cuts are appropriate; for larger structures, such as the kidneys, thicker cuts will be suitable.

The degree to which structural detail needs to be explored. In this respect, the **spacing** between adjacent tomographs (pivot heights) is also considered. For more complex structures (anatomically or pathologically) thinner layers at closer intervals will tend to be needed.

The inherent contrast of the structure being radio-

graphed. Here, the relationship is simple: the thinner the cut, the lower the image contrast. Thus, while bony structures can be tomographed to show thin layers, there is a limit to the narrowness of cut through soft-tissue structures, which will preserve useful image contrast.

Film exposure technique

The single-film, or sequential technique

This allows the fullest range of intensifying screens to be used, and enables each tomograph to be accurately identified.

The simultaneous multisection technique

This method, illustrated by Figure 50, lessens the waste of potential information represented by the image unsharpness of other layers, away from the pivot. Quite simply: the use of a series of films and intensifying screens separated by parallel

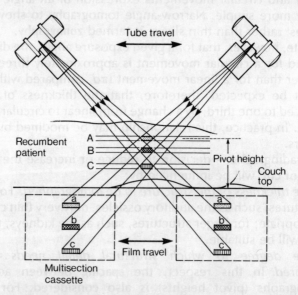

Fig. 50 The principle of simultaneous multisection tomography. Films spaced apart (a, b, c) record images of planes A, B, C. Note that the shaded areas are representative of the whole planes, and not just localised parts.

spacers in a multisection cassette will record a series of tomographs of corresponding layers through the body. Projected down to appropriate levels, the shadows of these different layers all 'move at the same speed'.

The limitations of this technique concern:

Consistent image density. Being positioned at varying distances from the X-ray tube, and because of attenuation within the upper parts of the multisection cassette, the radiation intensities impinging on each film and pair of intensifying screens, will differ — becoming less at lower levels within the cassette. To compensate, varying combinations of intensifying screens are used. The fastest combination is used for the lowest film, and there is a progressive reduction in speed towards the front of the cassette.

With such a multisection assembly, it is found that there is a minimum tube kilovoltage, below which consistency of image density cannot be maintained. On occasion, this may produce lower contrast than could be achieved with the single-film technique.

The use of varying screen speeds also causes photographic unsharpness to become more evident in the lower level tomographs.

Identification. A close look at Figure 50, shows that the spacing between the layers is exceeded by the separation between their images formed in the multisection cassette. This is the practical situation: films spaced 1 cm apart record tomographic layers which are less widely spaced. This occurs simply because of geometric magnification.

When a multisection cassette is used in place of a single cassette, it must be clearly known which of the cassette layers corresponds to the level of the single film — and, thus, to the indicated pivot height. Equipment varies: establishment of this relationship is essential for identifying the levels of individual tomographs.

The normal radiograph (data) identification equipment cannot be employed with films from a multisection cassette, and 'daylight' loading systems cannot be routinely used.

Advantages of the multisection technique include:

Speed: the time taken to expose a series of tomographs is significantly reduced.

Consistency of position: it is ensured that the patient is in a constant position for all the images within a simultaneously-exposed set.

Radiation protection: a significant reduction in the overall radiation dose to the patient, can be achieved by use of this technique.

Suggested exercise

— Students attending tomographic examinations should investigate why the various controllable factors are set at particular values, and why particular tube/film movements and exposure techniques are selected.

42

What is stereoradiography?

Principle

Normal human vision is binocular: the two eyes see objects from slightly different angles. These separate stimuli are combined by the brain into three-dimensional images: thus, the 'depth' of an object can be appreciated, as well as its 'height' and 'width'.

Single radiographic images show only two dimensions: they fail to demonstrate an object's 'depth'.

The principle of stereoradiography is summarised in Figure 51. Two separate radiographs of an object are exposed with the X-ray tube positioned, in turn, to the right and left. The radiographs are viewed simultaneously but each by its appropriate eye only, so that the eyes effectively, for viewing, replace the X-ray tube target, as it was positioned for the exposures.

The viewer is given the illusion of three-dimensional vision — but it is fixed: movement of the head from side to side cannot alter the angle of sight.

The technique of stereoradiography is not new. It was originally conceived in the nineteenth century to compensate for equipment deficiencies. Its place in modern techniques, where the practice of 'two projections at right angles' satisfies

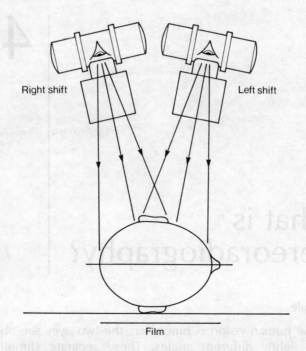

Right shift   Left shift

Film

Fig. 51 Stereoradiography: separate radiographs exposed when X-ray tube is positioned towards left and right are subsequently viewed separately by left and right eyes to convey the illusion of a three-dimensional image.

most situations, is not major. But students may occasionally encounter its use as an effective solution to the problem of showing three dimensions.

Some practical aspects

1. Immobilisation of the object is vital. If movement occurs during the interval while tube position and film are changed, the two stereoradiographs will not form a compatible pair. This risk imposes a limit on the possible applications of stereoradiography, unless a specialised, stereo X-ray tube is used.

2. The distance or angle through which the X-ray tube is moved between exposures — the tube 'shift' — bears a relationship to the interpupillary distance, usually 6 cm.

3. In addition to its anatomical markers, each stereoradiograph must be clearly marked 'right shift' or 'left shift' and

the tube aspect must be indicated, so that viewing can be correct.

4. When viewing, the left eye must see only the 'left shift' radiograph; and the right eye only the 'right shift'.

5. Stereo viewing equipment (binoculars or a stereoscope) causes a left-to-right image reversal — 'lateral transposition' of each image. Accordingly, when mounted for viewing the radiographs must have their tube aspects facing the illuminated screens.

Suggested exercise

— If stereoscopic viewing equipment is available, students may be interested to expose a pair of stereoradiographs of a phantom — a dry skull, for example.

43

How should a student plan to learn a radiographic procedure?

Students' experiences vary. Sometimes a procedure is first encountered practically, in the X-ray department; another may receive theoretical coverage in the classroom before being observed in practice. Study of radiographic technique atlases and other books can be very helpful, either in previewing procedures or adding explanatory information to practical experience. All these are learning opportunities, through which students may find answers to their questions: how, where, when and why?

Most important, of course, is the acquisition of practical skills, through assisting at or actually performing radiographic procedures in the X-ray department. But this is best supported by systematic learning. For this purpose, students may find a basic framework useful, into which they can fit their acquired knowledge, until a complete picture has been built up.

The following is offered as a general model for adaptation to suit individual techniques and procedures:

1. *Indications and contra-indications*
2. *Special equipment requirements and accessories*
   a. essential
   b. desirable.
3. *Preparation of the patient*

    a. before arrival in the X-ray department
    b. immediately before the procedure.
4. *Contrast agent(s)*
    a. type
    b. quantity
    c. method and timing of introduction
    d. precautions.
5. *Programme of radiographic projections (including their timing)*
    a. routine
    b. alternative
    c. supplementary.
6. *General position of the patient for the examination*
7. *Details of individual projections*
    a. position of the patient
    b. position of the X-ray film
    c. direction and centring of the X-ray beam
    d. exposure factors:
        (i) tube kilovoltage
        (ii) tube current (mA)
        (iii) exposure time
        (iv) focus-film distance
        (v) focal spot size
        (vi) type of film and intensifying screens
        (vii) use of a secondary radiation grid.
8. *Radiation protection*
9. *After-care of the patient*

Suggested exercise

— Students might try out a framework of this type to summarise or plan their learning of radiographic procedures.

How are image artefacts caused?

An artefact is a feature of a radiographic image which is *not a natural part of the object*. If not recognised as such, an artefact might lead to an error in diagnosis. Usually, however, artefacts *are* identifiable. They may have a negligible effect on an image or they may cause a radiograph to need to be repeated. But in either case, an investigation must be undertaken (a) to discover its cause, and (b) to prevent its recurrence.

The shape, size and density of an artefact will give a clue to its cause but radiographers must be aware of the whole range of possible causes.

X-ray tube assembly

Only rarely will the cause of an artefact be found in the tube assembly. But a loose screw or particle of solder from the light beam collimator, for instance, could find its way into the path of the X-ray beam. In such a case, the artefact would be of low density and surrounded by a considerable penumbra (being very much closer to the tube than to the film).

The patient

Common causes include articles of jewellery and opaque articles of clothing or their fasteners. Splashes or stains of opaque substances (including contrast agents) can be found on a patient's X-ray gown, mattress, immobilisation pads or compression band. If so, the characteristic woven pattern is usually obvious.

The cassette and intensifying screens

Marks or blemishes in the front of a cassette or its use in an inverted position (back to front) may cause low-density artefacts. Similar effects will result from the presence of scratches or dirt on an intensifying screen's surface which reduce light emission from that area. A piece of paper accidentally trapped in a cassette will halve the image density in that area, which will (as with all opacities close to the film) have a sharp outline.

Film and processing

Emulsion deficiencies can usually be detected if the film's surface is viewed by reflected light. These may be handling scratches or manufacturing faults.

Marks from wet or greasy fingers are easy to identify, as are the small, crescent-shaped 'crimp' marks caused by buckling of a film (seen as low density against a dark background, or high density if against a lighter background).

Static electricity, generated by friction, causes either discrete 'star' marks or larger, branching 'tree' patterns of high density.

Fogging, by white light, safelight or X-rays can, in some cases, cause shadows which are hard to identify.

Automatic processors can be the source of a variety of artefacts, when they function incorrectly — through contamination, poor maintenance or 'wear and tear'.

Suggested exercise

— Students may find that there is a collection of radiographs showing artefacts — some commonplace, others bizarre — in the X-ray department or school. These may provide an interesting exercise in detection and serve as a caution to the consequences of carelessness.

45

What are the ideal conditions for viewing radiographs?

The effort taken to expose radiographs correctly should be equalled by the care taken in viewing them. Otherwise the full information offered by an image might not be appreciated. Correct orientation of a radiograph is important: left must be distinguished from right, and other markers — to indicate timing, for instance — must be observed. But care must also be taken to appreciate a radiograph's contrast. Three aspects of the viewing conditions need to be considered.

Illumination of the viewing screen

If a radiograph has been correctly exposed, the pattern of densities which forms the image should correspond exactly in area and relative values, with the radiation intensities transmitted through the patient. Image densities can be viewed correctly, only if the viewing screen is evenly illuminated to a suitable degree of brightness.

Even illumination will be ensured by the manufacturer, when the viewing screen is newly purchased. But with use, deterioration can occur in two respects: dust may accumulate on the screen (inside and outside) and on the fluorescent tubes and reflectors; and replacement fluorescent tubes might not be evenly matched for brightness and colour.

A viewing screen's degree of brightness is 'suitable' when it matches the radiograph's density values. Since these will vary for different radiographs, it is ideal for the screen light intensity to be adjustable. To cater for especially dense areas of an image, a separate, high intensity light should be available.

Exclusion of extraneous light

Ideally, the area of the illuminated screen should precisely match the area of the image. Otherwise 'extraneous' light shines around the edges of the radiograph, tending to dazzle the viewer and reduce appreciation of image detail.

Exclusion of this light may be achieved by adjustable shutters incorporated in the illuminator; alternatively, separate masks, made from black card, may be available.

Reduction of reflected light

The shiny surface of a radiograph will reflect light towards the viewer if the room is brightly lit. This reflected light supplements the light transmitted through the radiograph. It will appear to add more to the low levels transmitted through the denser parts of the image, than to the brighter areas. It will thus have the effect of reducing the observed, or 'subjective' radiographic contrast.

Ideally, a room or area designed for viewing radiographs should have low-level (or shielded) illumination to minimise reflection from the radiographs' surfaces.

Suggested exercises

— Students should become familiar with the routine procedure in the X-ray department, for maintaining the efficiency of the radiograph illuminators.
— Students should experiment to see the effects of correct and adverse viewing conditions on the subjective appearance of a single radiograph.

46

Why is specialised X-ray equipment necessary?

Although interpretations of the term 'basic' will vary, it is probably acceptable to describe:

— a ceiling-suspended or column-mounted rotating-anode X-ray tube
— a moderately-powered X-ray generator
— a tilting bucky couch with fluoroscopic facilities
— a vertical bucky or 'chest stand'

as a basic assembly of X-ray equipment. Many small hospitals have just such equipment — and its advantages lie in *versatility*. With it, most routine radiographic examinations can be performed. Its shortcomings lie in

— its limited ability to cope with some of the more complicated examinations
— its total inability to carry out 'specialised' procedures.

It may prove instructive, to analyse some of these shortcomings, as a means of recognising the need for specialised X-ray equipment.

Precision

There are limitations on the precision with which some exam-

190

inations can be performed, using basic equipment. Specialised projections of the skull can be very difficult to produce with consistency, unless a skull unit is available.

A tomographic attachment to a basic equipment assembly, is incapable of the precision which a purpose-designed unit can achieve.

Even a modest intra-oral dental X-ray unit scores over general-purpose equipment, in terms of its accuracy.

Safety and comfort of the patient

The amount of handling an injured or very ill patient has to undergo, is lessened by the use of a simple 'floating-top' X-ray couch.

The problem of 'fitting the patient to the equipment' rather than manoeuvring the equipment around the patient, is acute when badly-injured casualty patients need to be radiographed. Specialised 'accident systems', particularly those employing an 'isocentric' principle, overcome this problem.

The patient's comfort and technical accuracy are both increased for techniques such as mammography, when specialised equipment is used.

Speed

This has two aspects: exposure repetition and patient throughput.

For some examinations of the cardiovascular system, rapid serial exposure equipment and an appropriate high-powered generator are essential. The more routine technique of chest radiography, although within the resources of basic equipment, is performed at an otherwise unattainable speed by a specialised chest unit, incorporating exposure automation and a film processing unit.

Summary

An X-ray department's range of equipment reflects the clinical demands which it needs to meet, in terms of both its variety and frequency. A balance is seen between the versatility of general equipment and the greater precision, safety and speed which, *for selected purposes*, specialised equipment can offer.

Suggested exercise

— Students might survey the range of equipment installed in the X-ray department (and enquire about plans for its development) to appreciate the relative contributions each makes to the overall service.

47

How do X-ray tube overload prevention devices operate?

Student radiographers will have seen that restrictions are imposed on the combinations of tube kilovoltage, current (mA) and exposure time which can be used, when exposure factors are selected. These can be traced to the problem presented by the heat which accompanies production of X-rays.

For each of its focal spot sizes an X-ray tube has a maximum safe rate at which heat may be produced. This rate reflects aspects of the tube's design, and is expressed (for particular voltage supply waveforms) in terms of kilovoltage, current and time. If an unsafe combination were to be exceeded, 'overload' damage to the X-ray tube would occur and its working life would be unduly shortened.

An overload prevention device translates selected kV, mA and exposure time values into their anticipated, combined anode heating effect. If this remains within safe limits, the exposure is allowed to go ahead. If not, exposure is blocked by a safety interlock until the radiographer has readjusted the selected values, to drop the heating rate.

The limits are, to some extent, arbitrary: they are set with due regard for the need to give the X-ray tube a satisfactory working life. They also carry the presumption that a suitable interval (the few minutes required for the patient to be repositioned and the film changed) will occur between exposures. In this regard, they are open to misuse: if the interval is not observed, overheating of the tube's anode may occur.

This weakness is remedied by the incorporation of a thermal sensor device within the X-ray tube which monitors anode temperature. With this refinement, overload prevention effectively allows an X-ray tube a safe and acceptably long working life.

Suggested exercise

— Students should, by experiment, see how, for a fixed kVp, the maximum permitted mA value falls, as the total selected milliampere-seconds value is increased. The results for both focal spots of an X-ray tube should be compared.

Related studies

X-ray tube design and rating; safety interlocks; types of overload prevention device.

48

How does an automatic exposure timer work?

If the densities recorded on a radiograph are outside an acceptable range, a repeat radiograph may be necessary — with all the accompanying expense, waste of time and increased radiation dose for the patient. Miscalculation of the required exposure for a radiograph — the milliampere-seconds value — is mainly responsible for such repeats.

Ideally, a radiographer would like to be able to terminate an exposure after the radiographic density has increased to the required level. This is impossible to achieve directly: not only is the X-ray film hidden from view, it shows no densities until it has been processed!

But such a monitoring process *can* be achieved indirectly by a logical arrangement of facts:

1. Radiation densities are produced by processing. If processing is reliably standardised, the densities are proportional to the exposures received by the film.

2. If film and intensifying screen speeds are known, radiographic densities can be controlled by exposure.

3. But this exposure is *not* a value 'set' by the radiographer: it is the radiation emerging from the object after it has been moderated by attenuation.

4. If this *transmitted* radiation is monitored, radiographic densities *can* be controlled, independently of the varying

attenuation which 'large' and 'small' objects produce. In other words, the unknown factor — the radiopacity of the object — can be eliminated as a source of trouble when radiographs are exposed.

Now to be considered, is the question of how this can be achieved. Two methods are available — each linked to a property of X-radiation: its ability to cause either *fluorescence* or *ionisation*.

Phototimers

If the X-ray equipment concerned incorporates a fluorescent screen, the light from this screen can be used to time radiographic exposures. Length of exposure is inversely related to screen brightness. Thus, a 'thin' patient — producing minimal attenuation — will allow the screen to remain relatively bright, and the exposure will terminate rapidly. A 'larger' patient will reduce screen brightness and cause the exposure to be prolonged.

Ionisation-chamber timers

The insertion of a thin, radiolucent ionisation chamber between the patient and the film, allows transmitted radiation to be measured, without casting an unwanted shadow on the radiograph.

The controls provided for the radiographer offer a choice of radiographic densities. Tube kilovoltage and current are set, as usual. Then, selection of a particular density 'programmes' the timer to terminate the X-ray exposure when an appropriate quantity of radiation has been detected by the ionisation chamber. Note that correlation of exposure to density must take account of film and intensifying screen speed, and processing efficiency. The controls may also include some form of moderation with regard to tube kilovoltage, and the 'manual' exposure timer on the X-ray control panel must be set to a slightly excess value.

When using an automatic exposure timer of this type, radiographers need to pay careful attention to the relative locations of patient and ionisation chamber, and to X-ray beam collimation.

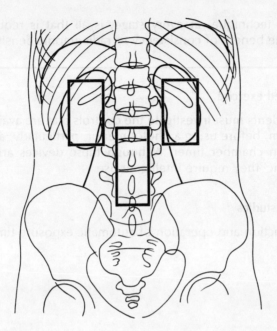

Fig. 52 Automatic exposure timing: separate ionisation chambers are provided to match representative anatomical areas, for determining radiographic density.

It is impractical for the area of the ionisation chamber to match the whole object being radiographed. Instead, it is common for three smaller alternative chambers to be available. Figure 52 illustrates such a situation. The central chamber will be appropriate to small field and centralised structures (skull, spine) while the lateral chambers will be preferable for chest and abdomen radiographs.

The important relationship to establish is that the chosen area is representative of the whole radiograph and that a given density in this area will imply correct exposure of the *whole* image.

X-ray beam collimation is required to be standardised, since an ionisation chamber's response will be influenced by lesser or greater amounts of scattered radiation, and it will interpret exclusion from the primary field, as being a very large patient!

The above points concerning the use of an automatic exposure timer are *precautions*, not disadvantages. Careful radiographic technique, at every stage, is all that is required to bring the benefit of consistency to radiographic densities.

Suggested exercise

— Students must investigate the controls that are available to them, before using a phototimer or, particularly, an ionisation chamber timer. Although these devices are 'automatic' they require intelligent use.

Related studies

Construction and operation of automatic exposure timers.

49

How can student radiographers help to maintain the safety and efficiency of X-ray equipment?

As users of X-ray equipment, student radiographers have a responsibility to themselves, their patients, and to all colleagues, to ensure that faulty operation of any equipment is identified, reported and dealt with, as a matter of urgency.

Identification of faults

When encountering any equipment for the first time, a student radiographer must learn thoroughly how to operate it, with accuracy and safety. Attention to this, in fact, reduces the likelihood that faults will occur, since a proportion of them are 'operator-induced'. It also forms a basis from which to be able to identify faulty operation or performance.

If a fault of any description is observed or suspected, a student's first action must be to ensure safety. Relevant points include electrical isolation of the equipment and temporary removal of the patient, while the fault is investigated. Once this has been attended to, a report must be made to an appropriately senior member of staff. The responsibility has then been passed on, but the student may still be involved in the investigation of the fault, and may be able to assist in its correction.

Unless a student encounters a unique fault, there is likely to be a laid-down investigation procedure. It will be regretted that the fault has occurred but, without this experience, students' education will be lacking — since, at some time in the future, it may be a responsibility of theirs, as qualified radiographers, to instigate the required procedure.

Implications of faults

To underline the importance of attending to them promptly, it may be helpful, briefly, to consider the consequences of neglect.

The seriousness of faults which threaten electrical and mechanical safety of equipment is obvious. Their effects could be fatal.

Any fault which implies an increased radiation hazard for the patient must be treated as an emergency. Otherwise, the need for maintaining radiation protection is neglected.

Minor faults can develop into major faults. Toleration of a seemingly insignificant problem can allow deterioration to occur with all its increased consequences.

All equipment breakdowns cause inconvenience, delay and expense. The cost of repairs and servicing is invariably high — but it is only relevant if considered against the total value of the equipment and its installation, and the expense of having to undertake more extensive repairs, later.

Suggested exercises

— All X-ray equipment is supplied with illustrated instruction manuals and leaflets. Students should read these, to learn the safest and most efficient methods of operation.
— Students must become familiar with the procedures required in their X-ray departments, in the event of equipment breakdowns. A study must be made of the various tests which can be carried out to verify suspected faults.
— It may prove interesting (and, in developing a sympathetic attitude towards the equipment, useful) for students to compile a price list of some items of X-ray equipment together with other, everyday commodities. Suggested inclusions are: a secondary radiation grid, a colour tele-

vision set, an X-ray tube, a car, a mobile X-ray set and a house.

Related studies

Regulations and instructions governing safe and accurate operation of equipment. Tests procedures to check performance of equipment and verify suspected faults.

50

In what ways can radiographers take care of their patients?

Radiographers take care of their patients by attending to *things that matter*.

To the radiographer, *technical competence* matters: high quality radiographic images, providing maximum diagnostic information from the minimum of radiation. Such professional standards are maintained in the patients' interests and are of high importance.

As their careers develop, radiographers will aim to acquire even more expertise. But preoccupation with technical skills must not overshadow the caring attitude which originally fostered the wish to become a radiographer.

To the patient, other things matter: it can be an illuminating experience for a radiographer to overhear a patient recounting a visit to the X-ray department.

It is quite normal for patients to regard the staff of an X-ray department (including students) as collectively responsible for everything that happens. It is right that this should be so; pride in the department should not be confined to one or two: staff should share a common pride and, if problems arise, a common responsibility.

Lack of communication accounts for much of what is seen as lack of care. Patients are normally very tolerant but they do like to be told what is going on. Having made the effort to attend punctually for an appointment, for instance, a patient deserves the courtesy of an explanation for *any* delay.

Sometimes it is just the *effort* the radiographer is seen to make which gives the patient comfort. A cup of tea, a magazine to read, an extra blanket, a window closed or opened are all simple, caring gestures which count for a lot, to a patient.

But perhaps the best insights radiographers have into appreciating a patient's priorities are gained on the occasions when *they themselves* are patients. Then, quite unsuspected things — tone of voice, smartness of a uniform — can be significant.

The list of points for students to think about is very long, indeed. Too long to be included in a book.

Index